AF326701

ISBN: 978-1-970503-06-7

Published by: WDP Publishing

Printed in: USA

For permission or inquiries:

✉ wendy@wdp-publishing.com.

First Edition, 2025

ABOUT THE AUTHOR

WENDY D. PALMER

She is a registered nurse, medical case manager, and writer with more than three decades of experience in trauma, emergency, acute care, and interventional radiology nursing. Throughout her career, she has worked closely with patients and families navigating complex medical conditions, giving her a deep understanding of both the science of health and the human experience behind every diagnosis.

Living with Parkinson's disease for over twenty years, Wendy brings a rare and powerful perspective to her writing—one that blends clinical expertise with lived experience. Her journey with a neurodegenerative condition has shaped her passion for brain health, cognitive resilience, and quality of life, prompting extensive research into how lifestyle choices, emotional well-being, and purposeful living can support the brain over time.

In addition to her professional background, Wendy's work is informed by profound personal experiences that have deepened her empathy, insight, and advocacy. These experiences have strengthened her commitment to helping others understand the brain not only as a biological organ, but as the center of identity, memory, and meaning.

Through her writing, Wendy seeks to translate complex medical and neurological concepts into accessible, compassionate guidance. Her goal is not simply to extend life, but to support mental clarity, dignity, and fulfillment at every stage of living, especially in the face of chronic illness or neurological change.

Wendy lives in Kentucky with her husband and family, where she continues to write, research, and advocate for greater awareness of brain health and neurological conditions.

ABSTRACT

In an era where science and technology have extended human lifespans beyond what our ancestors could imagine, "Secrets of the Centenarians" bridges the gap between ancient wisdom and modern breakthroughs in longevity research. This comprehensive guide explores how life expectancy has evolved from merely 30-40 years in medieval times to today's potential of living past 100. By examining the world's Blue Zones and incorporating cutting-edge scientific research, we'll uncover the secrets of those who've mastered the art of aging gracefully. This book offers a practical blueprint for extending not just your lifespan, but your healthspan - the period of life where you remain active, vibrant, and cognitively sharp.

TABLE OF CONTENTS

INTRODUCTION

In the quiet villages of Okinawa, the mountainous regions of Sardinia, and the bustling communities of Loma Linda, California, extraordinary individuals are defying our conventional understanding of aging. These centenarians - people who have lived beyond 100 years - aren't just surviving; they're thriving, often maintaining active, purposeful lives well into their second century. Their secrets, passed down through generations and now validated by modern science, hold the key to not just extending our years, but enriching the quality of those additional decades.

Just two centuries ago, the average human lifespan was a mere 35 years. Disease, harsh living conditions, and limited medical knowledge created a ceiling on human longevity that seemed insurmountable. Today, we stand at an unprecedented moment in human history, where living past 90 or even 100 is increasingly common in certain regions of the world. This remarkable transformation isn't just about medical advances - it's about understanding and implementing the wisdom of cultures that have long known the secrets to living longer, healthier lives.

Through my years of research and experiences interviewing centenarians across the globe, I've discovered that the path to exceptional longevity isn't found in a single breakthrough or miracle cure. Instead, it lies in the careful integration of ancient wisdom with modern scientific understanding. The practices that have sustained these long-lived communities - from their dietary habits and movement patterns to their social structures and stress-management techniques - offer profound insights that can be adapted for our contemporary world.

Perhaps most striking is how these centenarians maintain their cognitive vitality. In an age where neurodegenerative diseases pose increasing challenges, traditional practices for maintaining brain health have gained

new relevance. From the memory-enhancing techniques of ancient Greek scholars to the mindfulness practices of Buddhist monasteries, these time-tested methods are now being validated by modern neuroscience, offering hope for maintaining mental acuity throughout our extended lifespans.

This book is more than just a collection of longevity secrets - it's a practical guide to implementing the world's most effective aging-well practices in your own life. We'll explore how traditional fermentation techniques enhance gut health and immunity, how ancient movement practices maintain mobility and strength, and how time-tested stress management methods can help navigate our modern world's unique challenges.

As we delve into these practices, you'll meet remarkable individuals who embody these principles - like Maria from Sardinia, who still tends her garden at 102, and Dr. Zhang from China, who combines traditional Chinese medicine with modern geriatric care to help others achieve optimal aging. Their stories, along with cutting-edge research and practical implementation strategies, will show you how to create your own longevity blueprint.

The journey to exceptional longevity isn't about following a rigid set of rules or completely overhauling your lifestyle. Instead, it's about understanding and selectively adopting the most effective practices from various cultures, adapting them to fit your life, and gradually building habits that can support your health for decades to come. Whether you're in your 30s and looking to establish healthy aging practices early, or in your 60s and seeking to optimize your wellbeing, the principles in this book offer a roadmap to living longer, healthier, and more vibrantly.

As we begin this exploration together, remember that the goal isn't just to add years to your life, but to add life to your years. The wisdom of centenarians teaches us that longevity isn't just about duration - it's about quality, purpose, and the joy of living well at any age. Let's discover how we can apply their time-tested secrets to create our own path to exceptional health and longevity.

CHAPTER 1

The Evolution of Human Longevity

From Short Lives to Centenarian Potential

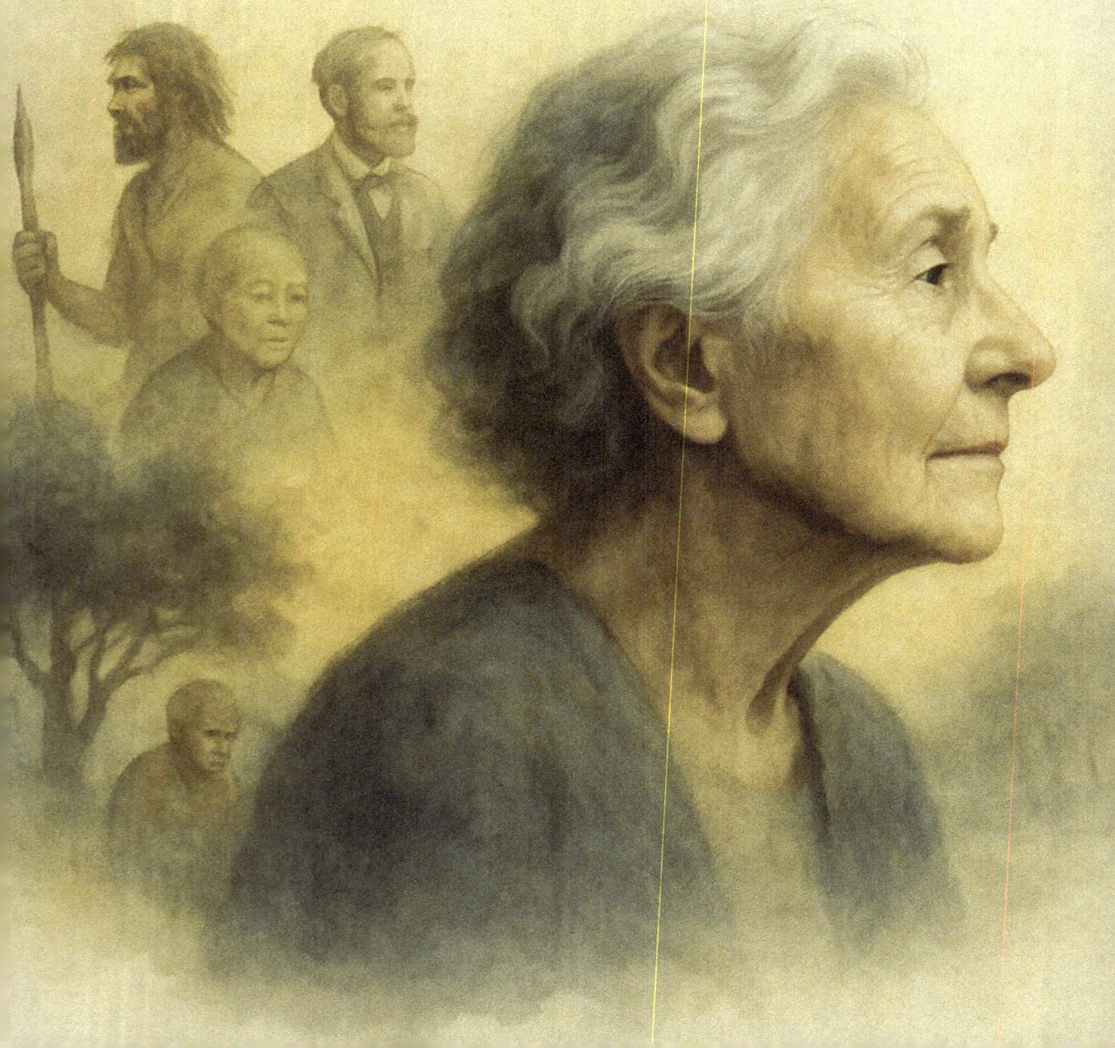

Thoughout most of human history, reaching the age of 40 was considered a remarkable achievement, with infectious diseases, harsh living conditions, and limited medical knowledge creating a ceiling on human lifespan. Today, we stand at an unprecedented moment in human evolution, where living past 100 is not only possible but increasingly common in certain regions of the world, marking a dramatic shift in our species' relationship with time and aging. This remarkable transformation in human longevity is a testament to our species' resilience and adaptability, as well as our growing understanding of the factors that influence healthy aging. The dramatic increase in life expectancy can be attributed to several key developments: advances in medical science, improved sanitation, enhanced nutrition, and perhaps most importantly, our deepening comprehension of how lifestyle choices impact longevity.

In the mountains of Sardinia, I met Aria, a vibrant 103-year-old woman who became my window into understanding the evolution of human longevity. Her family history reads like a timeline of humanity's progress in extending life expectancy. She shared stories passed down through generations about her great-grandmother, who died at just 45 - an age considered 'old' in the late 1800s. Aria's own journey through the 20th century paralleled humanity's increasing lifespan. She witnessed the introduction of antibiotics that saved her children from diseases that had claimed her siblings, experienced the transformation of food systems from subsistence farming to global nutrition, and embraced both traditional wisdom and modern medical advances.

What struck me most about Aria was how she embodied the

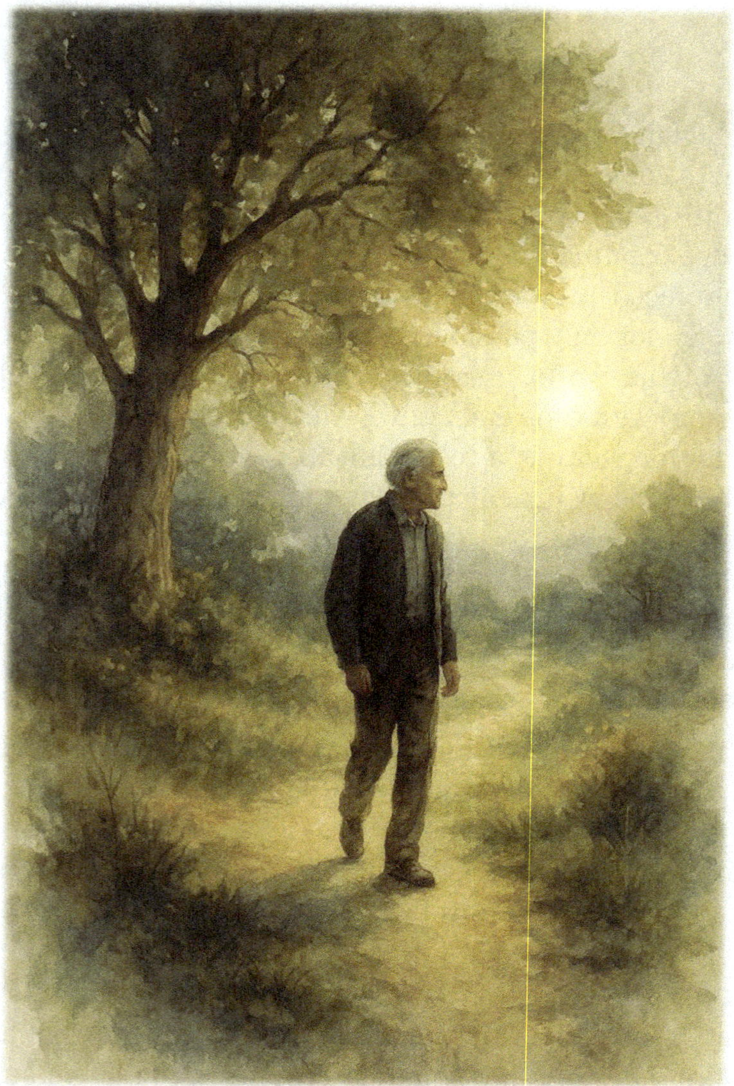

perfect bridge between old and new - she maintained the traditional Sardinian lifestyle that had served her ancestors well, while selectively incorporating modern medical care when needed. Her daily routine included tending her garden using ancient agricultural techniques, preparing meals following centuries-old recipes, and walking the same mountain paths her ancestors had traversed. Yet she also understood the value of regular health check-ups and appropriate medication.

Through Aria's story, we witness the remarkable evolution of human longevity - not just in numbers, but in the quality of life possible at advanced ages. Her experience demonstrates how we can harness both ancient wisdom and modern science to unlock our full longevity potential. It's a testament to how far we've come and a glimpse of what's possible when we combine the best of traditional practices with contemporary medical knowledge.

As we delve deeper into the secrets of human longevity, we'll explore how various factors - from lifestyle choices to environmental conditions - have shaped our ability to live longer, healthier lives. We'll examine how modern science validates many traditional practices while offering new insights into the mechanisms of aging. Most importantly, we'll discover practical ways to apply these lessons to our own lives, regardless of our current age or circumstances.

The journey to understanding human longevity is both a look back at where we've come from and a vision of where we're heading. It's a story of triumph over the historical limitations that once kept human life expectancy remarkably short, and a roadmap for pushing those boundaries even further. As we explore this fascinating evolution, we'll uncover actionable insights that can help each of us maximize our own longevity potential.

Historical Perspectives on Human Lifespan: From Hunter-Gatherers to Industrial Revolution

The story of human longevity is a remarkable journey through time, marked by dramatic shifts in how long people could expect to live. Archaeological evidence reveals that our hunter-gatherer ancestors faced significantly shorter lifespans than we enjoy today, though not necessarily for the reasons many assume. While life expectancy at birth during the hunter-gatherer period typically ranged from 21 to 37 years[1,3], this figure was heavily skewed by extremely high infant and childhood mortality rates. Those who survived their early years often lived much longer than commonly believed.

Research by anthropologists Gurven and Kaplan revealed a fascinating truth about our ancestors - among adults in hunter-gatherer societies, the most common age at death fell between 68 and 78 years[2,3,4]. This finding contradicts earlier assumptions that few people lived past 40 in prehistoric times. In fact, if individuals survived to age 15, about 64% could expect to reach at least 45 years of age[1,3]. These statistics paint a more nuanced picture of early human longevity, suggesting that our biological potential for long life has deep evolutionary roots.

The transition to agricultural societies, beginning around 10,000 BCE, brought unexpected challenges to human health and longevity. Contrary to what many might expect, the shift to farming initially led to poorer nutrition and increased exposure to infectious diseases[5]. As populations became more densely packed in settled communities, new health challenges emerged. The close proximity of humans to domesticated animals and larger community sizes created perfect conditions for the spread of diseases, while less varied diets often resulted in nutritional deficiencies[5].

Life expectancy remained relatively stable through ancient and medieval times, with most societies seeing average lifespans at birth between 20 and 35 years[2,3]. However, these figures again largely reflected high infant mortality rates rather than an absence of older individuals. Those who survived childhood in ancient Greece, Rome, or medieval Europe could often expect to live into their 50s or 60s, though reaching such ages was far from guaranteed.

The real revolution in human longevity began with the Industrial Revolution and subsequent advances in public health. Improved sanitation, better nutrition, and eventually medical breakthroughs like vaccines dramatically reduced childhood mortality. By 1900, life expectancy at birth in Western Europe and North America had reached 40-50 years - a significant increase from previous eras. This upward trend has continued into modern times, driven by continued advances in medical science, nutrition, and our understanding of factors that influence healthy aging.

Perhaps most striking is how different causes of death were in earlier times compared to today. In hunter-gatherer societies, about 70% of deaths resulted from infectious diseases, while 20% were due to violence or accidents, and only 10% stemmed from degenerative diseases[1]. This distribution stands in sharp contrast to modern societies, where chronic and degenerative conditions have become the primary causes of mortality.

Understanding this historical perspective helps us appreciate both how far we've come and what we can learn from our ancestors. While we've largely conquered many of the infectious diseases that once limited human lifespan, we now face new challenges related to lifestyle diseases and aging-related conditions. The key to further extending human longevity may lie in combining the best of modern medical science with lessons from our past - including the importance of physical activity, social connections, and varied, nutrient-rich diets that characterized many traditional societies.

The Public Health Revolution: How Sanitation and Medicine Transformed Longevity

The transformation of human life expectancy through advances in public health and medicine stands as one of humanity's greatest achievements. In the mid-1800s, the average person could expect to live only 40 years[6], with many succumbing to diseases we now easily prevent or treat. The primary culprits behind these shortened lifespans were poor sanitation, contaminated water supplies, and the unchecked spread of infectious diseases that ravaged communities with devastating regularity.

The first major breakthrough came through understanding the critical importance of clean water and proper waste management. The introduction of modern sewage systems and water treatment facilities in major cities during the 19th century marked a turning point in public health. These innovations dramatically reduced the spread of cholera, typhoid, and other waterborne diseases that had previously claimed countless lives[10]. In London, for example, the implementation of proper sewage systems in the 1860s led to a significant decline in cholera outbreaks that had regularly devastated the city's population.

The discovery and widespread implementation of vaccination programs represented another pivotal moment in extending human longevity. Beginning with Edward Jenner's smallpox vaccine, immunization has saved countless lives and contributed significantly to increasing life expectancy. The subsequent development of vaccines for diseases like polio, measles, and diphtheria transformed these once-deadly threats into preventable conditions[6,7]. This vaccination revolution continues today, with modern medical science providing protection against an ever-growing list of infectious diseases.

Perhaps one of the most significant medical breakthroughs came with the discovery of antibiotics. When Alexander Fleming discovered penicillin in 1928, he opened the door to treating bacterial infections that had previously been death sentences. The widespread availability of antibiotics by the 1940s marked a new era in medicine, where previously lethal infections could be cured with a simple course of treatment[7,8]. This development alone added years to average life expectancy and saved countless lives.

The establishment of public health agencies and surveillance systems further accelerated improvements in population health. These organizations implemented widespread health education programs, monitored disease outbreaks, and coordinated responses to health threats. Their work in promoting preventive care and healthy lifestyle practices has been crucial in extending not just lifespan, but also healthspan - the period of life lived in good health.

Nutrition has played an equally vital role in this revolution. The understanding of essential nutrients, vitamins, and balanced diets has helped eliminate many deficiency diseases that once shortened lives. Access to varied, nutritious food became more widespread, though this remains a challenge in many parts of the world. The combination of improved nutrition with advances in sanitation and medicine created a powerful foundation for longer, healthier lives[7].

Today, we stand at a fascinating juncture in the history of human longevity. While the rapid gains in life expectancy seen in the 20th century have begun to plateau in developed nations, we're witnessing the emergence of a new phenomenon - the centenarian population. Research indicates that we may be approaching what scientists call a "soft limit" for average life expectancy - around 89 years for women and 83 years for men[8]. However, this doesn't mean we've reached the absolute ceiling of human potential for long life.

The public health revolution has fundamentally altered our relationship with mortality. Where our ancestors once considered reaching 40 a remarkable achievement[9], we now regularly see people living well into their 80s and 90s. This transformation represents more than just additional years of life - it's a testament to human ingenuity and our capacity to overcome seemingly insurmountable challenges through scientific understanding and public health initiatives.

As we look to the future, the focus is shifting from merely extending life to ensuring those additional years are lived in good health. Modern public health challenges center around chronic diseases, lifestyle factors, and the aging process itself. The lessons learned from the public health revolution - the importance of preventive care, the value of systematic approaches to health challenges, and the power of combined scientific and social initiatives - continue to guide our efforts in promoting longevity and well-being in the 21st century.

Nutritional Evolution: From Survival to Optimal Health

The journey of human nutrition mirrors our species' remarkable evolution from mere survival to the pursuit of optimal health and longevity[11] [12]. Throughout most of human history, our ancestors faced a constant struggle to secure enough calories for basic survival, with food choices dictated by availability rather than nutritional value[12]. This fundamental challenge, combined with limited understanding of nutrition and hygiene, contributed significantly to historically shorter lifespans.

In prehistoric times, our hunter-gatherer ancestors relied on a diverse but unpredictable diet of wild plants, fruits, nuts, roots, and animal proteins[12]. While this diet was surprisingly nutrient-rich when food was abundant, periods of scarcity were common and often deadly. The agricultural revolution, beginning around 10,000 BCE, brought more reliable food sources but paradoxically led to less dietary diversity and new nutritional challenges. Early farming communities often suffered from malnutrition due to over-reliance on a limited number of staple crops.

The industrial revolution marked another pivotal shift in human nutrition, introducing processed foods, refined sugars, and flours on an unprecedented scale[12]. While these innovations helped eliminate widespread hunger in developed nations, they also gave rise to new health challenges. The modern "nutrition transition" has seen traditional, nutrient-rich diets replaced by processed, energy-dense foods - a change that correlates directly with increasing rates of chronic diseases and shortened healthspans.

However, research into the world's longest-lived populations reveals a fascinating counterpoint to these trends. In the "Blue

Zones" - regions with unusually high concentrations of centenarians - we find communities that have maintained traditional dietary patterns while selectively incorporating modern nutritional knowledge[11] [12]. These populations share remarkable commonalities in their approach to food and nutrition.

One of the most striking features of centenarian diets is their emphasis on plant-based nutrition[11] [12]. Blue Zone communities typically derive the majority of their calories from vegetables, legumes, whole grains, and fruits, with minimal processed foods. This pattern provides not just essential nutrients but also vital compounds that support cellular repair and reduce inflammation - key factors in extending both lifespan and healthspan.

Moderation emerges as another crucial principle in longevity-promoting diets. In Okinawa, Japan, the cultural practice of "hara hachi bu" - eating until 80% full - has been linked to reduced metabolic stress and improved cellular health[12]. This approach, combined with natural caloric restriction through primarily plant-based diets, appears to activate longevity pathways in the body.

The role of traditional food preparation methods cannot be overlooked. Fermentation, a preservation technique used for millennia, has been shown to enhance nutrient bioavailability and support gut microbiota diversity. Modern research confirms that a healthy gut microbiome is essential for both physical and cognitive health, potentially explaining why fermented foods feature prominently in many centenarian diets.

Perhaps most importantly, these dietary patterns exist within broader cultural contexts that support longevity. Meals in Blue Zone regions are typically social events, shared with family and community members[12]. This practice not only promotes slower, more mindful eating but also provides regular social interaction - a factor increasingly recognized as crucial for cognitive health and longevity.

The evolution of our understanding of nutrition has revealed that optimal health requires more than just adequate calories or even a balanced diet[12]. It demands attention to food quality, preparation methods, and the social context of eating. Modern science continues to validate many traditional dietary practices while offering new insights into how nutrition influences aging at the cellular level.

As we look to the future, the challenge lies not in choosing between traditional wisdom and modern science, but in combining both to create sustainable dietary practices that support longevity. The lessons learned from centenarian populations provide a valuable blueprint for this integration, showing how traditional dietary wisdom can be adapted to meet contemporary nutritional needs while promoting both healthspan and lifespan.

The Role of Modern Medicine and Technology in Extending Life

The dramatic extension of human life expectancy stands as one of modern medicine's greatest achievements. While our ancestors in the early 1900s could expect to live only 40-50 years, today's medical advances have pushed average lifespans well beyond 80 in many developed nations[11]. This remarkable transformation stems from multiple breakthroughs that have fundamentally changed our relationship with mortality and aging.

The story of Jeanne Calment, who lived to the extraordinary age of 122 years and 164 days, exemplifies the profound impact of modern medicine and technology on human longevity[11][13]. Born in 1875, she lived through an era that saw the introduction of antibiotics, vaccines, advanced surgical techniques, and countless other medical innovations that would have been unimaginable in her youth[13]. Her record-breaking lifespan demonstrates the remarkable potential for human longevity when medical advancement, genetics, and lifestyle factors align optimally.

The control of infectious diseases marks one of medicine's most significant contributions to longevity. Through vaccination programs and antibiotics, illnesses that once decimated populations - such as smallpox, polio, and bacterial infections - have been either eradicated or rendered largely treatable[11]. This transformation alone has saved countless lives and added decades to average life expectancy.

Cardiovascular care represents another crucial area where modern medicine has extended lifespans. The development of medications for managing hypertension, cholesterol-lowering statins, and advanced surgical interventions like stents and bypass procedures has dramatically improved survival rates for heart disease patients[11]. These innovations, combined with better diagnostic tools such as MRI and CT scans, allow for earlier detection and more effective treatment of potentially fatal conditions[11].

The rise of personalized medicine and genetic engineering presents exciting possibilities for further extending human longevity. Technologies like CRISPR offer potential solutions for correcting genetic disorders and possibly slowing aging processes at the cellular level[11]. Meanwhile, regenerative medicine and stem cell research suggest future possibilities for repairing or replacing aging organs[11], potentially pushing the boundaries of human lifespan even further.

Artificial intelligence has emerged as a powerful tool in modern medicine's arsenal against aging and disease. By accelerating drug discovery, optimizing treatment protocols, and predicting health risks, AI is helping healthcare providers make more informed decisions and deliver more effective treatments[11]. This technological revolution extends beyond traditional medical settings, with smartphones and wearable devices now enabling individuals to monitor their health metrics and make lifestyle adjustments that support longevity[14].

However, the extension of human lifespan through modern medicine raises important ethical considerations. While centenarians are becoming more common, debates continue about whether there exists a biological limit to human longevity, regardless of medical advances[11]. Additionally, questions of quality versus quantity of life become increasingly relevant as we push the boundaries of human lifespan[11].

Perhaps most critically, access to these life-extending medical innovations remains uneven across global populations. While some benefit from cutting-edge treatments and technologies, others lack access to even basic healthcare services, creating stark disparities in longevity potential between different regions and socioeconomic groups[11].

Looking ahead, the future of longevity medicine appears both promising and challenging. As we continue to unlock the mysteries of aging through genetic research, artificial intelligence, and regenerative medicine, the potential for extending human lifespan grows. Yet this potential must be balanced against ethical considerations and the imperative to ensure equitable access to life-extending medical innovations across all populations.

The role of modern medicine and technology in extending life represents more than just a triumph of science - it reflects humanity's persistent quest to understand and optimize our biological potential. As we continue to push the boundaries of human longevity, the integration of traditional wisdom with cutting-edge medical innovation may hold the key to not just longer lives, but healthier, more fulfilling ones as well.

Blueprint for Centenarian Potential: Combining Ancient Wisdom with Modern Science

The quest for longevity has evolved dramatically from our ancestors' struggle for survival to today's scientific pursuit of optimal aging. While historical records show most people lived only 40-50 years in the early 1900s, we now regularly witness individuals reaching their centennial year with vitality and purpose[11]. This remarkable transformation reflects both our growing understanding of the aging process and our ability to combine ancient wisdom with modern scientific insights.

The dramatic increase in human longevity isn't merely a product of modern medicine - it represents a complex interplay between traditional knowledge and scientific advancement. Research into Blue Zones, regions with the highest concentrations of centenarians, reveals that these communities have naturally integrated ancient practices with selective modern innovations[13]. Their success in producing centenarians stems from what scientists now call the "Power 9" - nine lifestyle habits that combine age-old wisdom with contemporary understanding of health and longevity[13].

Perhaps most striking is how Blue Zone communities demonstrate the effectiveness of traditional dietary patterns. Their primarily plant-based diets, emphasis on moderate portions, and practice of eating until only 80% full align perfectly with modern research on caloric restriction and longevity[13]. These ancient eating patterns, now validated by scientific studies, show how traditional wisdom often anticipates modern discoveries about health and aging.

The role of movement in longevity presents another compelling example of ancient wisdom meeting modern science. While our ancestors engaged in constant, natural movement through daily activities, today's research confirms that this pattern of regular, moderate physical activity is more beneficial for longevity than intense but sporadic exercise[11] [13]. This understanding has led to a shift in modern fitness recommendations, moving away from purely gym-based workouts toward incorporating more natural movement throughout the day.

Social connections and community bonds, long emphasized in traditional societies, have now been scientifically validated as crucial factors in longevity[11]. Modern research confirms that strong social networks and a sense of purpose - elements naturally embedded in traditional communities - significantly impact both lifespan and healthspan. The Japanese concept of "ikigai" (a reason for being) and similar traditional philosophies about life purpose have been shown to correlate with extended longevity and better health outcomes[13].

Modern science has also validated many traditional stress management practices. Ancient techniques like meditation, mindful breathing, and community gatherings are now understood to reduce chronic inflammation and improve cellular health - key factors in aging[14]. These practices, when combined with modern stress-reduction techniques, create a powerful toolkit for managing the psychological challenges of contemporary life while promoting longevity.

The blueprint for centenarian potential emerges from this synthesis of old and new. It involves understanding that while genetics play a role (accounting for 20-30% of longevity)[11] [13], the majority of factors influencing lifespan are within our control. This empowering reality suggests that by adopting a combination of time-tested practices and evidence-based modern approaches, we can significantly influence our potential for reaching a healthy old age.

The case of Jeanne Calment, who lived to 122 years and 164 days, exemplifies this synthesis[11] [13]. Her lifestyle combined traditional elements like regular olive oil consumption and maintaining a positive attitude with modern medical care and adaptation to changing times. Her extraordinary longevity demonstrates how traditional wisdom and modern science can work together to extend not just lifespan, but healthspan.

Creating a personal blueprint for centenarian potential requires understanding and implementing key elements from both traditional wisdom and modern science. This includes adopting a predominantly plant-based diet[11] [13], engaging in regular natural movement[11] [13], maintaining strong social connections[11], finding purpose in daily life[11], and managing stress through both ancient and modern techniques[14]. It also means taking advantage of modern medical advances while respecting the wisdom of traditional health practices.

The path to exceptional longevity isn't about choosing between ancient wisdom and modern science - it's about creating a synergy between the two. By understanding how traditional practices align with scientific research, we can develop more effective strategies for extending both lifespan and healthspan. This integrated approach offers our best chance at not just living longer, but maintaining vitality and purpose throughout our extended years.As we conclude this journey through the remarkable evolution of human longevity, it's clear that our potential for living longer, healthier lives has never been greater. From the harsh realities of our ancestors, who often succumbed to infectious diseases and environmental challenges before reaching 40, to today's growing population of vibrant centenarians, the story of human longevity is one of triumph over seemingly insurmountable obstacles.

The dramatic increase in life expectancy we've witnessed isn't merely a product of medical advancement - though innovations in sanitation, vaccination, and disease treatment have played crucial roles. Rather, it represents our species' extraordinary ability to learn from both ancient wisdom and modern science. Through Aria's story, we've seen how traditional practices can harmoniously coexist with contemporary medical knowledge, creating a powerful foundation for extended longevity.

Our exploration of historical perspectives has revealed that while our ancestors faced significant challenges to longevity, they also developed sophisticated systems of health maintenance that continue to inform our understanding of wellness today. The public health revolution transformed our relationship with mortality, while advances in nutrition have helped us move from mere survival to optimal health.

Perhaps most encouraging is our growing understanding of the factors within our control. While genetics play a role in longevity, research shows that lifestyle choices, environmental factors, and daily habits significantly influence our potential for healthy aging. The combination of traditional wisdom and modern science offers us an unprecedented opportunity to not just extend our lives, but to maintain vitality and purpose throughout our years.

As we look to the future, the blueprint for centenarian potential becomes clearer. It involves embracing both time-tested practices and evidence-based innovations, maintaining strong social connections, engaging in regular physical activity, and nurturing our mental and emotional well-being. The story of human longevity continues to unfold, offering hope and practical guidance for those seeking to optimize their own health and longevity.

In the chapters ahead, we'll delve deeper into specific practices and principles that can help you develop your own longevity blueprint. We'll explore how to adapt ancient wisdom for modern life, harness the power of nutrition and movement, and maintain cognitive vitality throughout the years. The journey to exceptional longevity isn't about choosing between old and new - it's about creating a synergy that supports optimal health and wellness at every stage of life.

Remember, our prehistoric ancestors who survived to adulthood often lived into their 60s and 70s, suggesting that human longevity isn't a modern phenomenon but rather a natural potential we're now learning to fully realize. By understanding and applying the lessons from both our past and our present, we can work toward not just longer lives, but lives rich in health, purpose, and vitality.

As we move forward, let this chapter serve as a foundation for understanding how far we've come in our quest for longevity, and more importantly, how much potential still lies ahead. The secrets of the centenarians aren't just in their genes or their medical care - they're in the daily practices, lifestyle choices, and wisdom accumulated over generations. By embracing these lessons and adapting them to our modern context, we can each work toward optimizing our own longevity potential.

CHAPTER 2

Blue Zone Secrets

Universal Principles from Earth's Longest-Living Communities

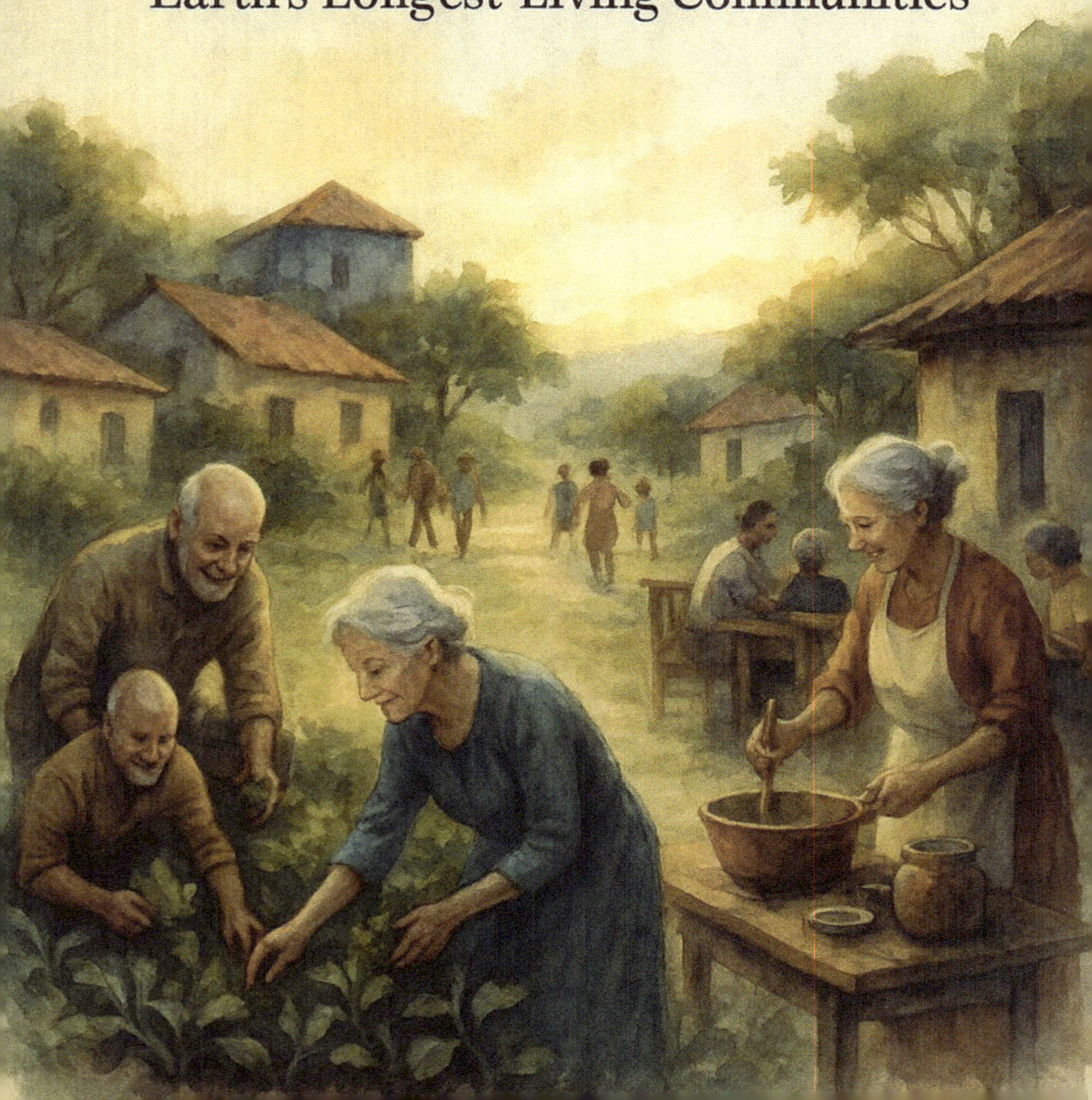

In the sun-drenched villages of Sardinia and the tropical islands of Okinawa, remarkable communities have unlocked the secrets to extraordinary longevity, consistently producing centenarians who remain vibrant and engaged well past their hundredth birthday. These Blue Zones, as they've come to be known, share fascinating commonalities in lifestyle practices that transcend cultural and geographical boundaries, offering us a blueprint for extending not just our lifespan, but our healthspan. These remarkable pockets of exceptional longevity have captured the imagination of researchers and health enthusiasts worldwide, offering living proof that extended life expectancy isn't just about surviving - it's about thriving well into our later years. The Blue Zones represent more than just geographical locations; they embody a harmonious blend of lifestyle practices that have proven successful across generations and cultures.

What makes these regions particularly fascinating is how their inhabitants have naturally maintained practices that modern science now validates as crucial for longevity. From the mountainous villages of Sardinia to the tropical paradise of Okinawa, these communities share striking commonalities in their approach to diet, physical activity, social connections, and stress management. They've discovered - or perhaps preserved - what many of us in the modern world are desperately trying to reclaim: a balanced, purposeful way of living that promotes both quantity and quality of life.

Their secrets aren't found in expensive supplements or complicated exercise regimens. Instead, they lie in simple, sustainable practices that have been woven into the fabric of daily life. These communities demonstrate that longevity isn't achieved through extreme measures but through consistent, wholesome habits maintained over a lifetime.

I witnessed this truth firsthand during my time with Dakota, a 35-year-old software engineer from Seattle who had taken a sabbatical to live in various Blue Zones and document their practices. In Okinawa, she immersed herself in the local lifestyle, joining a moai (social support group) of elderly women who gathered daily for tea and conversation. Initially skeptical about how these traditional practices could fit into her modern life, Dakota was transformed by her experience. She witnessed firsthand how the Okinawan elders maintained their gardens well into their 90s, practiced tai chi at dawn, and gathered for community meals filled with laughter and purpose.

The most profound impact came from observing their approach to stress management - a stark contrast to her former lifestyle of deadline-driven anxiety. Upon returning home, Dakota restructured her life around Blue Zone principles, creating a modern moai with her neighbors, converting her balcony into a small vegetable garden, and prioritizing natural movement over gym sessions. Within six months, her blood pressure normalized, her sleep improved, and most importantly, she found a sense of purpose and community she hadn't known she was missing. Her story illustrates how Blue Zone wisdom can be successfully adapted to contemporary life, bridging the gap between ancient practices and modern reality.

As we delve deeper into the secrets of these remarkable regions, we'll uncover how their various practices interweave to create a tapestry of well-being that transcends cultural boundaries. Through understanding these universal principles, we can begin to craft our own path to longevity, adapting their time-tested wisdom to our modern context while maintaining the essence of what makes these practices so effective.

In the following sections, we'll explore each of the key elements that make the Blue Zones unique - from their plant-forward nutrition and natural movement patterns to their strong social bonds and stress-management techniques. More importantly, we'll discover how to translate these practices into actionable strategies that work within the constraints of our busy, modern lives.

Plant-Forward Nutrition: The 95/5 Rule of Blue Zone Diets

One of the most striking features across all Blue Zone regions is their remarkable adherence to what researchers have termed the "95/5 Rule" of nutrition - a dietary pattern where approximately 95% of daily calories come from plant-based sources, with only about 5% derived from animal products[15][17]. This principle stands in stark contrast to modern Western diets, yet it consistently emerges as a cornerstone of exceptional longevity.

In these remarkable communities, the dinner plate tells a story of agricultural wisdom passed down through generations. Vibrant vegetables, hearty whole grains, and protein-rich legumes take center stage, while meat appears more as a garnish than a main course[17]. This dietary pattern isn't a modern health trend but a traditional way of eating that has sustained these populations for centuries.

The science behind this approach is compelling. Studies conducted in Blue Zones show that this plant-forward diet contributes significantly to lower rates of heart disease, diabetes, and certain cancers[16]. The abundance of antioxidants, fiber, and essential nutrients found in plant foods appears to create an optimal environment for cellular health and longevity.

In Sardinia, for instance, the traditional diet centers around whole grain sourdough bread, garden vegetables, and legumes, with small portions of pecorino cheese and occasional meat[15]. Okinawans historically derived the vast majority of their calories from sweet potatoes, green vegetables, and soy products, with fish served in small amounts as a complement to their plant-based meals[15].

What's particularly noteworthy is how this dietary pattern supports not just physical health but cognitive function as well. The high levels of antioxidants and anti-inflammatory compounds found in plant foods help protect against neurodegenerative diseases, while the limited intake of processed foods and refined sugars helps maintain stable blood sugar levels - a key factor in brain health[15].

The 95/5 rule isn't about strict limitation but rather about abundance - an abundance of fresh, whole foods that provide sustained energy and nutrition[15] [17]. In Blue Zone communities, meals are built around beans, greens, whole grains, and tubers, with fruits and nuts as regular components[15]. These foods are typically prepared simply, often using just a handful of ingredients and traditional cooking methods that preserve their nutritional value[15].

Fermented foods play a significant role in this dietary pattern, appearing regularly in forms like tofu, pickled vegetables, and sourdough bread[15]. These foods not only add variety to meals but also support digestive health and nutrient absorption - factors that contribute to overall longevity.

Perhaps most importantly, this way of eating isn't viewed as a diet in these communities - it's simply their way of life. Food is celebrated, shared with family and friends, and deeply connected to local traditions and seasonal rhythms[15] [16]. Meals are social events, not just fuel for the body, contributing to both physical and emotional well-being.

The 95/5 rule demonstrates that a predominantly plant-based diet doesn't mean complete elimination of animal products. Rather, it suggests a thoughtful balance where small amounts of animal foods complement and enhance a foundation of plant-based nutrition[17]. This approach has proven sustainable across generations, supporting not just longevity but quality of life well into advanced age[15][17].

In practical terms, adopting this principle doesn't require radical change but rather a gradual shift toward more plant-based meals. It might mean starting the day with whole grain porridge topped with fruits instead of processed cereals, or making beans and vegetables the stars of dinner plates while treating meat as a condiment rather than the main attraction[15].

This dietary wisdom from the Blue Zones offers a powerful lesson for our modern world: the path to longevity doesn't require expensive superfoods or complicated dietary rules. Instead, it points us toward a simple, sustainable way of eating that has stood the test of time[15], supporting not just individual health but the vitality of entire communities.

Movement as Medicine: Natural Physical Activity Patterns

In the world's longest-lived communities, movement isn't relegated to an hour at the gym or a weekend workout - it's an integral part of daily life that flows as naturally as breathing. Unlike our modern approach to exercise, which often involves structured routines and dedicated fitness sessions, Blue Zone inhabitants demonstrate that natural, consistent physical activity woven into the fabric of everyday living holds the key to extraordinary longevity[11][18].

This wisdom stands in stark contrast to our contemporary sedentary lifestyle, which research has identified as a leading risk factor for chronic disease and early mortality. In Blue Zones, people don't "exercise" in the conventional sense - instead, their environments and daily routines necessitate regular movement. Whether it's Sardinian shepherds traversing hilly terrain, Okinawan elders tending their gardens, or Nicoya Peninsula residents walking long distances and working the land by hand, movement is purposeful and persistent throughout life.

The biological benefits of this approach are profound and well-documented. Continuous, low-intensity physical activity improves cardiovascular health, lowers blood pressure, and helps maintain muscle mass and bone density well into advanced age. Perhaps most significantly, this natural movement pattern supports healthy glucose metabolism and reduces the risk of type 2 diabetes[11], while simultaneously stimulating brain health and enhancing cognitive resilience.

Dan Buettner, the pioneering Blue Zones researcher, observed that "the world's longest-lived people don't pump iron, run marathons, or join gyms. Instead, they live in environments that nudge them into moving without thinking about it." This insight reveals a crucial distinction between exercise as we know it and the movement patterns that support exceptional longevity.

In these communities, physical activity persists across the lifespan, with elders remaining active participants in society well into their 90s and beyond. The concept of retirement from physical activity is virtually non-existent - instead, work and movement adapt but rarely cease. This continuous engagement helps maintain not just physical health but also cognitive function and social connections, creating a powerful synergy for longevity.

The variety and moderation inherent in these natural movement patterns are equally important. Activities are diverse - walking, gardening, manual crafts - providing balanced physical stimulus without the risk of overuse injuries common in modern exercise regimens. While the intensity remains modest, the total volume of movement is high and sustained, creating optimal conditions for longevity.

Perhaps most importantly, movement in Blue Zones is purpose-driven and socially integrated. Physical activity isn't performed for its own sake but as a byproduct of meaningful tasks: growing food, caring for family, maintaining homes, and engaging with community. This integration of purpose with movement creates a sustainable pattern that can be maintained throughout life, unlike the often short-lived motivation behind many modern exercise programs.

The World Health Organization emphasizes that physical inactivity ranks among the leading risk factors for global mortality, underscoring the importance of integrating movement into daily life. The evidence from Blue Zones suggests that the solution isn't found in expensive gym memberships or intense workout routines, but in creating environments and lifestyles that make natural movement unavoidable and meaningful.

This understanding offers valuable lessons for our modern world. While we may not all be able to live as shepherds or farmers, we can incorporate principles of natural movement into our daily lives. Simple changes like walking for transportation, taking stairs instead of elevators, or maintaining a garden can help replicate the movement patterns that have supported exceptional longevity in Blue Zone communities for generations.

Social Connections and Community Bonds

Among the most powerful determinants of longevity discovered in Blue Zone communities is the strength of social connections and community bonds. Research led by Dr. Julianne Holt-Lunstad revealed that social isolation poses a mortality risk comparable to smoking or obesity, highlighting how crucial meaningful relationships are to our survival and well-being[19].

In these remarkable longevity hotspots, social interaction isn't an afterthought - it's woven into the very fabric of daily life[20]. The Okinawan practice of moai exemplifies this beautifully, where individuals belong to lifelong social groups that provide emotional, financial, and physical support throughout their lives[20]. These traditional support systems ensure that no one faces life's challenges alone, creating a buffer against stress and fostering resilience well into advanced age.

The power of these social bonds extends beyond emotional comfort - they have measurable impacts on physical health. Studies have shown that individuals with strong social connections have a 50% higher likelihood of survival compared to those with weaker social ties[20]. This remarkable finding underscores how our relationships quite literally shape our longevity.

In Blue Zone communities, multi-generational households remain common, creating continuous opportunities for meaningful interaction across age groups[20]. This arrangement ensures that elders remain active participants in family life, sharing wisdom while receiving care and support. The constant engagement helps maintain cognitive function and provides a sense of purpose that proves vital for healthy aging.

Daily intimate contact with family and friends is prioritized in these long-lived communities[19]. Unlike modern societies where social interactions often take a backseat to work and other commitments, Blue Zone inhabitants make time for regular visits and shared meals. These aren't just pleasant social occasions - they're investments in longevity, creating the emotional connections that help sustain health and vitality.

Community participation extends beyond family bonds through social groups centered around shared purposes, beliefs, or hobbies[20]. Whether through religious communities, volunteer organizations, or interest-based groups, these connections provide additional layers of support and meaning. The sense of belonging and life satisfaction that comes from such engagement has been shown to enhance both physical and mental well-being.

Perhaps most importantly, these communities understand that social connection is a two-way street. Longevity experts have found that helping others is as beneficial as receiving support, creating a virtuous cycle that strengthens community bonds while combating isolation[19]. This mutual support system ensures that everyone has opportunities to both give and receive care, fostering a deep sense of interdependence and shared purpose.

The implications for modern life are clear - we must prioritize and nurture our social connections with the same dedication we give to diet and exercise[20]. This might mean creating our own versions of moai, scheduling regular family meals, or joining community groups that align with our interests and values. While our social structures may differ from traditional Blue Zone communities, the fundamental need for strong social bonds remains unchanged.

In an age where technology often substitutes for face-to-face interaction, the wisdom of Blue Zones reminds us that virtual connections cannot fully replace the profound benefits of direct human contact[20]. The challenge for modern societies is to create environments and opportunities that facilitate meaningful social interaction, recognizing that our relationships are not just pleasant additions to life - they are essential ingredients for longevity.

As we seek to incorporate Blue Zone principles into our lives, strengthening social connections may be among the most challenging yet rewarding changes we can make[20] [19]. It requires intentional effort to build and maintain relationships in our fast-paced world, but the research is clear - investing in our social bonds pays dividends in both the quality and quantity of our years.

Purpose-Driven Living: The Power of 'Ikigai' and 'Plan de Vida'

Among the most profound discoveries from Blue Zone research is the vital role that purpose plays in extending not just lifespan, but healthspan. Two remarkable frameworks for purpose-driven living have emerged from these longevity hotspots: the Japanese concept of 'Ikigai' and the Costa Rican 'Plan de Vida.' These philosophies offer powerful insights into how a deep sense of purpose contributes to extraordinary longevity.

In Okinawa, Japan, ikigai represents far more than simply having a reason to wake up each morning - it embodies the intersection of what one loves, what one excels at, what the world needs, and what one can be compensated for[22] [23]. As documented by researchers Héctor García and Francesc Miralles in their groundbreaking study of Ogimi's centenarians, ikigai manifests as "the happiness of always being busy" - a state of continuous, joyful engagement with life that transcends Western notions of purpose[22] [21].

This concept is beautifully illustrated in the daily lives of Okinawan elders, who maintain active roles in their communities well into their 90s and beyond[22] [23]. Whether tending gardens, participating in community activities, or sharing wisdom with younger generations, these centenarians embody what García and Miralles describe as "having everything they need for a long and joyful journey through life"[22].

Paralleling ikigai is the Costa Rican concept of 'Plan de Vida' - literally "life plan" - found in the Nicoya Peninsula. Here, elders remain deeply integrated into family and community life, maintaining clear roles and responsibilities that provide an enduring sense of purpose. This integration ensures that older adults continue to contribute meaningfully to their families and communities, whether through work, childcare, or passing down traditional knowledge.

The science supporting these purpose-driven approaches is compelling. A landmark 2014 study published in Psychological Science demonstrated that individuals with a strong sense of purpose had significantly lower mortality risks, independent of other factors like age, gender, or emotional well-being. This research validates what Blue Zone communities have long understood - that purpose is not merely a psychological comfort but a biological imperative for longevity.

The practical application of these principles involves several key elements that have been distilled from Blue Zone observations. The "10 Rules of Ikigai," gathered from Okinawan elders, offer a framework for purpose-driven living that includes staying active without formal retirement, maintaining strong social connections, practicing moderation in eating (hara hachi bu), and cultivating a deep connection with nature[23].

Equally important is the emphasis both traditions place on continuous learning and adaptation. Unlike modern societies where retirement often marks a retreat from active engagement, Blue Zone elders embrace new challenges and responsibilities as they age[22] [23]. This ongoing growth mindset appears to support cognitive health while providing the sense of purpose that drives longevity.

Perhaps most significantly, both ikigai and Plan de Vida emphasize the importance of community contribution[22]. Whether through sharing harvested vegetables with neighbors in Okinawa or helping raise grandchildren in Nicoya, the act of giving to others creates a virtuous cycle of purpose and belonging. This stands in stark contrast to modern retirement paradigms that often isolate older adults from meaningful social roles.

The wisdom of these approaches offers valuable lessons for our modern world, where purpose often becomes disconnected from daily life. By understanding and adapting the principles of ikigai and Plan de Vida, we can create our own frameworks for purpose-driven living that support not just longer life, but a life filled with meaning and joy at every stage.

As we seek to incorporate these teachings into our lives, it's essential to remember that purpose isn't something we find once and hold onto forever. Rather, as demonstrated by Blue Zone centenarians, it's a dynamic force that evolves with us, providing continuous opportunities for growth, contribution, and connection throughout our lives.

Stress Management Through Traditional Practices

In the serene valleys of Ikaria and the tranquil villages of Okinawa, centenarians have mastered the art of stress management through practices that have been refined over generations[25] [24]. These traditional approaches to managing life's pressures stand in stark contrast to our modern world's often frantic pace, offering profound insights into how we can better navigate daily stresses while promoting longevity.

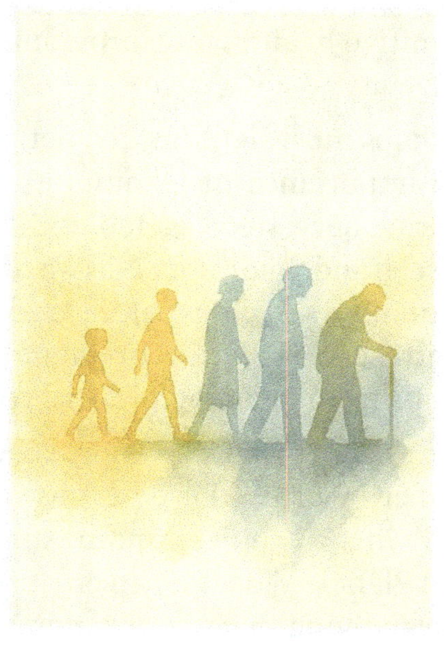

Research has consistently shown that chronic stress accelerates aging at the cellular level, contributing to inflammation, cardiovascular disease, and cognitive decline[25]. However, Blue Zone inhabitants have developed remarkably effective methods for maintaining emotional equilibrium, even in the face of life's inevitable challenges. Their approach isn't about eliminating stress entirely - rather, it's about developing resilient responses to life's pressures.

One of the most striking features of Blue Zone stress management is the practice of daily "downshifting" - intentional periods of relaxation or reflection that punctuate each day[25]. In Okinawa, this often takes the form of ancestor veneration and the pursuit of ikigai, while in Ikaria, residents engage in regular gardening and neighborly walks[25]. These aren't merely pleasant diversions; they're powerful stress-reduction techniques that have been validated by modern research.

The Adventist community in Loma Linda, California, offers particularly compelling evidence of how traditional stress management practices contribute to longevity. Their regular prayer and meditation sessions, combined with weekly Sabbath rest, provide structured downtime that allows for mental and physical recovery[25]. This systematic approach to stress reduction has been linked to their remarkably high life expectancy.

Dr. Thomas Perls and Margery Hutter Silver's research reveals that centenarians aren't necessarily people who avoided stress altogether, but rather those who developed exceptional coping mechanisms. As they note, "Centenarians are the Michael Jordans of stress management - the natural athletes of stress... It's not that they avoided stress... But they were people who seemed able to cope with their problems and tragedies and moved on with a positive outlook."[24]

In Sardinia, where some of the world's longest-lived men reside, stress management is deeply woven into the social fabric. Residents regularly gather for communal activities, sharing laughter and maintaining perspective through what researchers have termed "centenarian humor"[24]. This social approach to stress management creates a powerful buffer against life's challenges while strengthening community bonds.

The dietary habits in Blue Zones also play a crucial role in stress management. Their plant-based diets, rich in fruits, vegetables, legumes, and whole grains, provide natural anti-inflammatory and mood-stabilizing effects[25]. Meals are typically enjoyed slowly and in company, often accompanied by gratitude or prayer - practices that modern research confirms can significantly reduce stress levels.

Physical activity in Blue Zones serves a dual purpose - not only does it maintain physical health, but it also acts as a natural stress reliever. Unlike modern exercise routines, movement in these communities is naturally integrated into daily life through activities like gardening, walking, and household tasks[25]. This approach provides regular opportunities for both physical activity and mental decompression.

Perhaps most significantly, Blue Zone inhabitants maintain robust social support networks that serve as natural buffers against stress. Many live in multi-generational households or maintain close ties with extended family and neighbors[24]. This continuous social connection provides both emotional support and practical assistance during challenging times, creating a sustainable framework for stress resilience[26,24].

The wisdom of these traditional practices offers valuable lessons for our modern world, where stress-related health issues have reached epidemic proportions. By understanding and adapting these time-tested methods, we can develop more effective approaches to managing the unique pressures of contemporary life while promoting longevity and well-being.

As Margery Hutter Silver emphasizes, maintaining mental acuity through stress management is crucial for independence in later years: "Whether you retain your thinking abilities predicts whether you're going to be able to remain independent - much more than your physical condition. People can often compensate for physical disabilities with various devices and assistance, but if you don't have mental acuity, it's much more difficult."[24]

The universal principles of stress management found in Blue Zones - daily downshifting rituals, social connection, natural movement, mindful eating, and cultivation of adaptability - offer a comprehensive framework for building resilience. These practices, refined over generations and validated by modern research, provide a roadmap for managing stress while promoting the kind of robust longevity that characterizes the world's longest-lived communities[25,24,26].As we conclude our exploration of the world's Blue Zones and their extraordinary inhabitants, we find ourselves at a fascinating intersection of ancient wisdom and modern understanding. The practices we've uncovered in these longevity hotspots offer profound insights into how we can extend not just our lifespan - which has already increased dramatically from the mere 40-year average of our ancestors - but our healthspan, ensuring those extra years are lived with vitality and purpose.

The transformation from our shorter-lived past to our current potential for sustained longevity is remarkable. Where our ancestors faced challenges from infectious diseases, limited medical knowledge, and harsh living conditions, we now benefit from advances in healthcare, sanitation, and nutrition. However, the Blue Zones reveal that these modern advantages alone don't guarantee the exceptional longevity observed in their communities. Instead, it's the combination of these advances with time-tested lifestyle practices that creates the optimal conditions for long, healthy life.

Perhaps most striking is how the various elements we've explored - from plant-forward nutrition and natural movement to social connections and stress management - work in concert to support not just physical health, but cognitive vitality. The brain-healthy habits we've observed, from regular social engagement to purposeful activity and stress reduction, align perfectly with current neuroscience research on preventing cognitive decline. These communities demonstrate that maintaining mental acuity isn't about complex brain training programs, but about living in ways that naturally support cognitive health.

The wisdom of the Blue Zones also teaches us that longevity isn't about deprivation or rigid rules. Instead, it's about creating environments and habits that naturally support health and vitality. Whether it's the Okinawan practice of hara hachi bu (eating until 80% full), the Sardinian tradition of daily social interaction, or the Nicoyan emphasis on purpose through Plan de Vida, these practices show us how to make health-promoting choices feel natural and sustainable.

As we look to implement these lessons in our own lives, it's crucial to remember that we don't need to replicate Blue Zone practices exactly. Instead, we can adapt their core principles to our modern context while maintaining their essential benefits. Dakota's story demonstrates how these ancient practices can be successfully translated into contemporary life, creating positive changes that ripple through all aspects of health and well-being.

The Blue Zones remind us that extraordinary longevity isn't about finding a single secret or magic bullet. Rather, it's about embracing a holistic approach to life that nourishes body, mind, and spirit. These communities show us that the path to a longer, healthier life isn't found in extreme measures or the latest health fads, but in the wisdom of practices that have sustained human health and vitality for generations.

As we move forward, let's carry these lessons with us: the power of plant-based nutrition, the importance of natural movement, the crucial role of social connections, and the vital impact of purpose-driven living. These principles, when thoughtfully adapted to our modern lives, offer a roadmap not just to living longer, but to living better at every age. The Blue Zones stand as living proof that exceptional longevity is within our reach - not through revolutionary new discoveries, but through the timeless wisdom that has sustained human health and vitality for generations to come

CHAPTER 3

The Centenarian Diet

Mediteraneaan Wisdom Meets Japanese Longevity

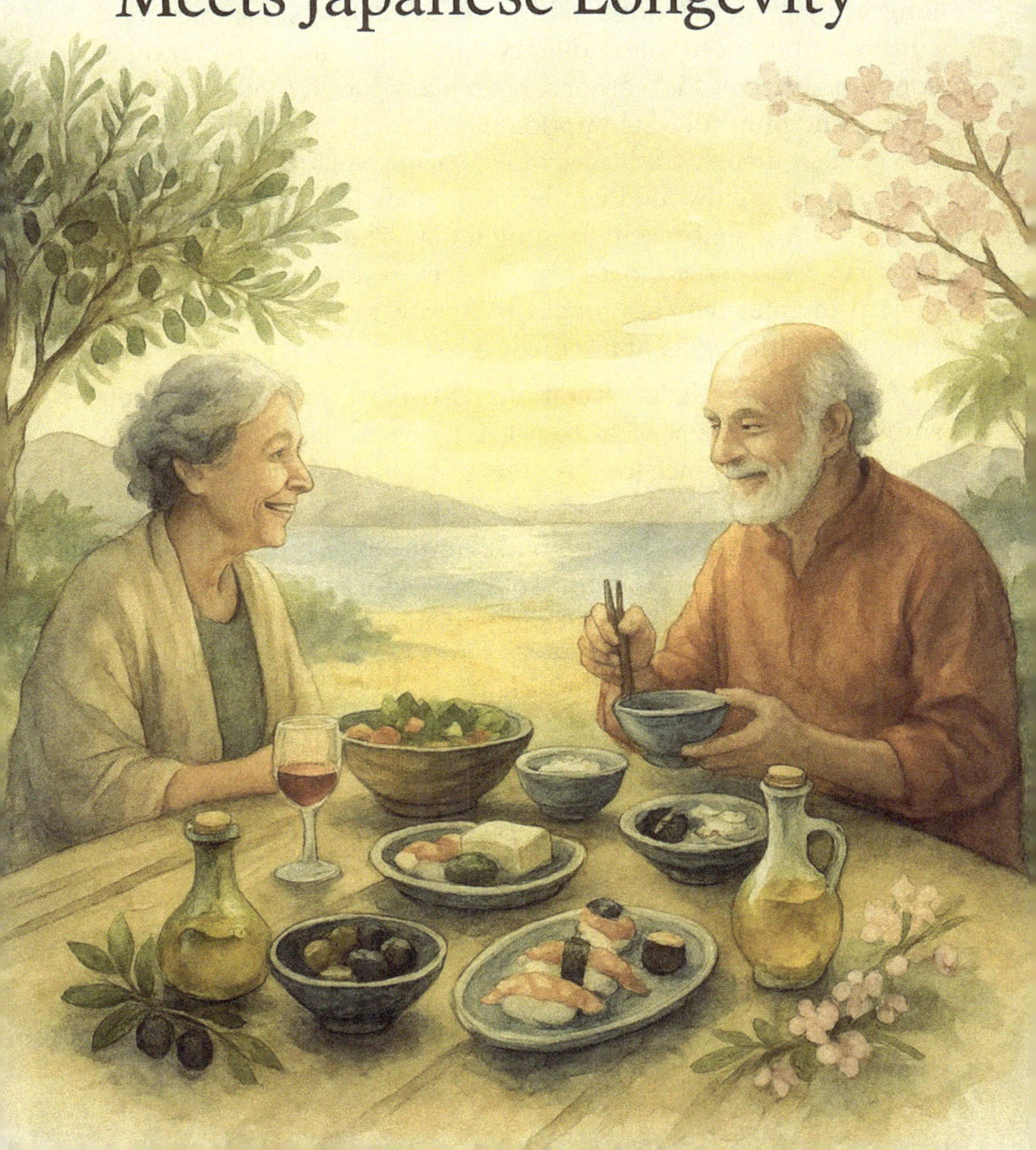

Beneath the azure skies of Crete and across the pristine shores of Okinawa, two distinct culinary traditions have independently evolved to support some of the world's longest-living populations. While separated by vast distances and cultural differences, these dietary approaches share remarkable commonalities in their emphasis on plant-based foods, seasonal eating, and mindful consumption patterns. The marriage of these two ancient dietary traditions offers us a powerful framework for understanding how food can become medicine - a concept both cultures have embraced for millennia. The wisdom of these practices has been validated by modern research, showing how their principles activate longevity pathways in our bodies and support healthy aging at a cellular level.

What makes these dietary traditions particularly fascinating is their emphasis on not just what to eat, but how to eat. Both cultures share a deep reverence for the ritual of dining, understanding that nourishment extends beyond mere calories and nutrients. They recognize that the way we approach our meals - with mindfulness, gratitude, and in the company of others - plays a crucial role in how our bodies process and benefit from the food we consume.

Perhaps one of the most striking features of both dietary traditions is their remarkable simplicity. Despite their sophistication in promoting health and longevity, the fundamental principles are straightforward: abundant plant foods, moderate protein primarily from fish and legumes, healthy fats from sources like olive oil and cold-water fish, and minimal processed foods. This simplicity makes these dietary approaches not just healthy, but sustainable and adaptable to modern life.

During my research into centenarian diets, I became familiar with Penelope, a Greek-Japanese fusion chef who had transformed her own health by combining both dietary traditions. At fifty-five, she had been diagnosed with high blood pressure and pre-diabetes, conditions that ran in her family. Determined to avoid the fate of her parents, who had struggled with chronic illness, Penelope embarked on a journey to explore her mixed heritage through food. She spent six months in her grandmother's village in Crete, learning to prepare traditional Mediterranean dishes, and another six months in Okinawa, studying local cooking methods. Through this immersive experience, she discovered how both cultures approached food not just as sustenance, but as medicine. She learned to combine Mediterranean olive oil with Japanese seaweed, to ferment vegetables using techniques from both traditions, and to practice the Okinawan principle of hara hachi bu while enjoying Mediterranean-style social meals. Within a year of implementing these combined dietary principles, her health markers had normalized, and she had lost twenty pounds without feeling deprived. Today, at sixty-five, Penelope teaches others how to blend these ancient dietary wisdoms into a practical, modern approach to eating. Her story demonstrates how the synthesis of these two longevity-promoting dietary traditions can create a powerful framework for optimal health.

As we delve deeper into these dietary traditions, we'll explore how their principles can be adapted to modern life without losing their essential benefits. We'll examine specific foods and preparation methods that have been scientifically proven to promote longevity, and discover how combining elements from both traditions can create a sustainable, enjoyable approach to eating that supports our health goals. Most importantly, we'll learn how to transform these ancient practices into practical, everyday habits that can help us live longer, healthier lives.

The Power of Polyphenols: Shared Plant-Based Foundations

At the heart of both Mediterranean and Japanese longevity lies a profound secret - the power of polyphenols, remarkable plant compounds that have been quietly supporting human health for millennia. These bioactive substances, found abundantly in both traditional diets, represent a fascinating convergence of ancient wisdom and modern scientific validation. While our ancestors may not have known the molecular mechanisms at work, they understood intuitively that certain plant-based foods held the key to vitality and longevity.

In both regions, the daily diet naturally incorporates a rich tapestry of polyphenol sources. The Mediterranean tradition embraces olive oil, laden with hydroxytyrosol and oleuropein, while the Japanese culture treasures green tea, brimming with powerful catechins[11] [18]. These dietary choices, passed down through generations, have proven remarkably prescient as modern research reveals the profound impact of polyphenols on cellular health and longevity.

The science behind polyphenols' effectiveness is compelling. These compounds act as powerful antioxidants, protecting our cells from oxidative stress and DNA damage - key factors in aging and age-related diseases[11]. They demonstrate remarkable anti-inflammatory properties, modulating the expression of inflammatory genes and cytokines that contribute to chronic diseases. Perhaps most intriguingly, certain polyphenols can cross the blood-brain barrier, offering neuroprotective benefits that may help explain the lower rates of cognitive decline observed in these populations.

The traditional diets of both regions share remarkable similarities in their approach to polyphenol consumption. Fresh, seasonal vegetables and fruits form the foundation of daily meals, ensuring a diverse spectrum of these beneficial compounds[11] [18]. Whole grains and legumes, rich in phenolic acids and other polyphenols, feature prominently in both cuisines. Even the traditional beverages - green tea in Japan and moderate red wine consumption in the Mediterranean - contribute significant polyphenol content to the diet.

Modern research has validated what these cultures have known through observation and tradition: polyphenol-rich diets correlate strongly with reduced rates of cardiovascular disease, diabetes, certain cancers, and cognitive decline[11]. The evidence suggests that these compounds work synergistically, creating a protective effect that extends beyond what any single polyphenol could achieve alone. This may explain why whole food sources, rather than isolated supplements, appear to offer the greatest benefits.

Perhaps most remarkably, polyphenols appear to influence our gut microbiota, fostering beneficial bacterial populations that contribute to overall health and longevity[18]. This emerging understanding of the gut-brain axis provides new insight into how traditional dietary practices may have supported not just physical health, but mental and emotional well-being as well.

The practical implications of this shared wisdom are clear. By incorporating a variety of polyphenol-rich foods into our daily diet - from colorful vegetables and fruits to herbs, spices, and traditional beverages - we can harness these powerful compounds for our own longevity[11][18]. The key lies not in dramatic dietary overhauls, but in returning to the simple, plant-forward eating patterns that have sustained health and vitality in these regions for generations.

Mindful Eating Practices and Portion Control Principles

In the tranquil mountain villages of Sardinia and the serene coastal towns of Okinawa, a profound wisdom surrounding the act of eating has been preserved through generations. These centenarian-rich regions share a remarkable approach to nourishment that extends far beyond the simple act of consuming food - they have mastered the art of mindful eating and portion control, practices that modern science now recognizes as crucial for longevity[11][18].

The Okinawan principle of "hara hachi bu" - eating until you're 80% full - stands as one of the most powerful examples of traditional portion control wisdom. This practice, deeply embedded in Okinawan culture, has been linked to their extraordinary longevity and low rates of age-related diseases[11][18]. Modern research validates this ancient wisdom, showing that moderate caloric intake can activate longevity pathways in our cells and support healthy aging.

In Mediterranean communities, similar principles manifest through different cultural practices. Meals are treated as sacred social occasions, with food served on smaller plates and eaten slowly over extended periods[11][18]. This natural pacing allows the body's satiety signals to function optimally, preventing overconsumption while fostering deeper connections with both food and family. The combination of mindful eating and social engagement creates a powerful synergy that supports both physical and emotional well-being.

The science behind these traditional practices is compelling. When we eat mindfully, our digestive systems function more efficiently, and we naturally consume fewer calories while deriving greater satisfaction from our meals[11][18][27]. Research shows that people who practice mindful eating and portion control tend to maintain healthier weights and experience lower rates of metabolic disorders - factors that significantly influence longevity.

These practices become particularly relevant when we consider how our relationship with food has evolved. In earlier times, food scarcity was a constant concern, and our ancestors developed sophisticated approaches to food that emphasized appreciation and moderation[11]. Today, in an era of abundance and rushed meals, these traditional practices offer a vital counterbalance to modern eating habits that often contribute to shortened lifespans.

Perhaps most intriguingly, mindful eating practices have been shown to support brain health, a crucial factor in healthy aging[11] [18]. The act of eating slowly and consciously engages multiple neural pathways, while proper portion control helps maintain optimal blood sugar levels - a key factor in preventing cognitive decline. The social aspects of traditional eating patterns also provide regular cognitive stimulation, contributing to mental resilience well into advanced age.

Implementing these principles in modern life requires thoughtful adaptation rather than rigid rules. The key lies in understanding the core wisdom: eat slowly, stop before fullness, minimize distractions during meals, and cultivate gratitude for food[11] [18]. Small changes, such as using smaller plates, taking time to appreciate each bite, and sharing meals with others, can help incorporate these centenarian practices into contemporary lifestyles.

The impact of these practices extends beyond physical health. Regular mindful eating helps reduce stress, improve sleep quality, and enhance overall well-being - all factors that contribute to longevity[11] [18] [27]. By treating meals as opportunities for nourishment rather than mere fuel stops, we tap into an ancient wisdom that modern science increasingly validates as essential for healthy aging.

In both Mediterranean and Japanese traditions, these practices are not viewed as restrictions but as natural expressions of respect for food and body[11] [18]. This positive approach makes these habits sustainable over a lifetime, contributing to the remarkable longevity observed in these regions. As we seek to extend our own healthspans, these time-tested practices offer valuable guidance for creating a healthier relationship with food and, ultimately, a longer, more vibrant life.

Sea-Based Nutrition: The Role of Fish and Seaweed

The azure waters surrounding Okinawa and the Mediterranean have long held secrets to longevity, providing abundant sources of fish and seaweed that have sustained centenarian populations for generations[11][18]. These marine treasures represent more than mere sustenance - they embody a sophisticated understanding of nutrition that modern science is now validating as crucial for extending both lifespan and healthspan.

In both regions, the consumption of fish and seaweed has been a cornerstone of dietary practices, with remarkable parallels in their approach to these nutrient-dense foods[11][18]. The Okinawan tradition of consuming small portions of fish daily, often accompanied by various seaweeds like wakame and kombu, mirrors the Mediterranean practice of regular fish consumption, particularly of small, oily varieties rich in omega-3 fatty acids. This dietary pattern has contributed significantly to the exceptional longevity observed in these regions[11].

The science behind these traditional practices is compelling. Fish provides essential omega-3 fatty acids, particularly EPA and DHA, which play crucial roles in brain health and cardiovascular function. These nutrients have been shown to reduce inflammation, support cognitive function, and protect against age-related decline. Similarly, seaweed offers an impressive array of nutrients, including iodine for thyroid health, unique polysaccharides with anti-inflammatory properties, and a rich spectrum of vitamins and minerals that support overall vitality.

Perhaps most intriguingly, the combination of fish and seaweed in traditional diets appears to create a synergistic effect. The iodine from seaweed supports optimal thyroid function, while the omega-3s from fish enhance the absorption of fat-soluble nutrients. Together, they provide a powerful nutritional foundation that supports both physical and cognitive longevity[11][18].

In Okinawa, where centenarians regularly consume both fish and seaweed, researchers have observed remarkably low rates of cardiovascular disease and cognitive decline[11]. The traditional practice of incorporating seaweed into daily miso soup and consuming small portions of fish has been linked to better thyroid function, reduced inflammation, and improved gut health - all factors that contribute to increased longevity.

The Mediterranean approach, while different in its specific preparations, shares similar principles[11]. Regular consumption of oily fishlike sardines and anchovies provides concentrated sources of omega-3s, while traditional fishing communities have long harvested and consumed local seaweeds, though to a lesser extent than their Japanese counterparts.

Modern research has validated these traditional practices, showing that populations consuming more fish and seaweed exhibit lower rates of cardiovascular disease, improved cognitive longevity, and reduced inflammation[11,18]. The unique compounds found in seaweed, such as fucoidan, have demonstrated immune-modulating properties, while the combination of high-quality protein and omega-3s in fish supports muscle maintenance and repair - crucial factors in healthy aging.

For those seeking to incorporate these longevity-promoting foods into their diet, the key lies in following the traditional wisdom of moderation and variety[11]. Small, daily portions of fish and seaweed, rather than occasional large servings, appear to provide the greatest benefits. Choosing smaller fish species helps minimize exposure to environmental toxins while maximizing nutritional benefits and incorporating various types of seaweed ensures a broad spectrum of beneficial compounds.

The practical application of this wisdom in modern life requires thoughtful adaptation. Simple practices like adding seaweed to soups and salads, choosing sustainably sourced small fish, and preparing these foods in traditional ways can help capture the longevity-promoting benefits observed in centenarian populations[11][18]. The goal is not to replicate these diets exactly, but to understand and apply their principles in a way that suits contemporary lifestyles while maintaining their essential benefits.

Fermentation Traditions and Gut Health

In the ancient valleys of Asia and the sun-drenched shores of the Mediterranean, our ancestors discovered a remarkable alchemy in the art of fermentation - a practice that would become one of humanity's most powerful tools for both food preservation and health promotion[11][18]. This time-honored tradition, which began as a necessity for survival, has emerged as a cornerstone of longevity in the world's healthiest populations. Modern science now validates what traditional cultures have known for millennia: fermented foods are not just sustenance, but medicine for the gut and, by extension, the entire body.

The science behind fermentation's health benefits is profound. When microorganisms transform ordinary foods through fermentation, they create a cascade of beneficial compounds that support our gut microbiota - the vast ecosystem of bacteria living within our digestive system. This process enhances the bioavailability of nutrients, produces beneficial short-chain fatty acids, and introduces living probiotics that can beneficially modulate our gut health. Research has shown that these mechanisms play crucial roles in reducing inflammation, supporting immune function, and potentially extending our healthspan.

In Mediterranean traditions, fermented foods take many forms, each contributing uniquely to gut health and longevity. Traditional yogurt, made from sheep or goat milk, delivers beneficial Lactobacillus and Bifidobacterium strains that support digestive health. Naturally fermented olives, rich in polyphenols and lactic acid bacteria, offer both anti-inflammatory benefits and support for microbial diversity. The region's traditional sourdough bread, fermented with wild yeasts and beneficial bacteria, provides better digestibility and a lower glycemic impact than conventional bread.

Japanese culture offers its own profound wisdom regarding fermented foods. Daily consumption of miso soup, rich in Aspergillus oryzae and beneficial bacteria, has been linked to better health outcomes in population studies. Natto, fermented soybeans processed with Bacillus subtilis, provides vitamin K2 and nattokinase, compounds associated with cardiovascular health. Traditional tsukemono (pickled vegetables) and naturally brewed soy sauce contribute additional layers of fermented nutrition to the daily diet.

The impact of these fermented foods on longevity is particularly evident in regions like Okinawa, where the traditional diet includes a daily array of fermented products[11] [18]. The Japan Gerontological Evaluation Study has found compelling correlations between fermented food consumption and improved cognitive function in older adults, while epidemiological research suggests that regular intake of fermented soy products is associated with lower rates of cardiovascular disease and certain cancers.

Perhaps most intriguingly, modern research is uncovering how fermented foods influence the gut-brain axis, suggesting these traditional foods may play a role in maintaining cognitive health and emotional well-being as we age. The short-chain fatty acids produced during fermentation have been shown to nourish colon cells, regulate immune function, and potentially protect against various age-related conditions.

In practical terms, incorporating these longevity-promoting foods into our modern diets requires thoughtful adaptation rather than dramatic overhaul. Starting with small daily portions of traditionally fermented foods - whether it's a bowl of miso soup, a serving of natural yogurt, or properly fermented vegetables - can help us capture the benefits observed in centenarian populations[11] [18]. The key lies in choosing unpasteurized, traditionally fermented options and combining them with fiber-rich plant foods to support optimal gut health.

The wisdom of fermentation traditions reminds us that some of our most powerful tools for health and longevity have been hiding in plain sight, preserved in the cultural practices of the world's healthiest populations. As we seek to extend our healthspan and support our gut health, these ancient practices offer a proven pathway to better health, validated by both centuries of traditional use and modern scientific understanding.

Seasonal Eating and Food Preparation Methods

In the world's longest-living communities, the rhythm of eating follows nature's own calendar - a practice that modern science increasingly recognizes as crucial for optimal health and longevity[11] [18]. This ancient wisdom, preserved in both Mediterranean and Japanese cultures, reveals a sophisticated understanding of how seasonal eating patterns and traditional food preparation methods support our body's natural cycles and promote healthy aging.

In Mediterranean regions, particularly in places like Sicily and Sardinia where centenarians thrive, the practice of eating seasonally isn't just a culinary preference - it's a way of life deeply embedded in cultural traditions[27]. Local markets burst with different offerings throughout the year: tender spring greens, sun-ripened summer tomatoes, autumn squashes, and winter citrus. This natural variety ensures a diverse spectrum of nutrients that support different aspects of health throughout the year.

Similarly, in Okinawa, where an extraordinary number of centenarians reside, seasonal eating patterns have been carefully documented by researchers studying longevity[11]. The traditional Okinawan diet shifts subtly with each season, incorporating specific local vegetables like bitter melon in summer and sweet potatoes through cooler months. This practice ensures optimal nutrition while maintaining harmony with the body's changing needs throughout the year.

The preparation methods in these longevity hotspots are equally significant. In Mediterranean communities, olive oil serves as the foundation of cooking, used both fresh and in gentle heating methods that preserve its heart-healthy compounds. Slow cooking and stewing predominate, techniques that not only enhance flavor but also improve nutrient bioavailability while minimizing the formation of harmful compounds associated with high-temperature cooking[27].

Japanese traditions offer complementary wisdom in food preparation. Their emphasis on raw and lightly cooked vegetables preserves vital nutrients and enzymes, while traditional fermentation practices - evident in foods like miso and tsukemono - enhance both preservation and nutritional value. The principle of hara hachi bu - eating until 80% full - demonstrates their sophisticated understanding of portion control and its impact on longevity[11 18].

Modern research validates these traditional approaches[11]. Studies show that seasonal produce often contains higher levels of beneficial compounds, including vitamins, minerals, and polyphenols, which may protect against age-related diseases. The traditional preparation methods used in both cultures have been linked to improved gut health, reduced inflammation, and better immune function - all crucial factors in healthy aging.

Perhaps most significantly, these seasonal eating patterns and preparation methods naturally support community bonds and social connections[11]. In both Mediterranean and Japanese cultures, the preparation and sharing of seasonal foods create opportunities for social interaction and cultural continuity - factors that research increasingly recognizes as vital for longevity.

The wisdom of these practices offers valuable lessons for modern life. While we may not have access to the exact same seasonal patterns as these longevity hotspots, we can adopt their core principles: choosing fresh, seasonal produce when available, employing gentle cooking methods that preserve nutrients, and maintaining connection to natural cycles through our food choices. These practices not only support physical health but also foster a deeper connection to the rhythms of nature that have sustained human health for generations.

In both traditions, the approach to food preparation and seasonal eating reflects a profound understanding of how our bodies interact with the natural world[11][18]. This wisdom, passed down through generations and now validated by scientific research, provides a valuable framework for those seeking to enhance their own health and longevity through mindful eating practices.As we conclude our exploration of the Mediterranean-Japanese dietary synthesis, we find ourselves at a remarkable intersection of ancient wisdom and modern science. The dietary practices we've examined - from the power of polyphenols to the art of fermentation - represent not just cultural traditions, but sophisticated systems for promoting longevity that have stood the test of time.

Through our journey, we've discovered how these dietary traditions have contributed to extending human lifespan far beyond what our ancestors could have imagined. In earlier centuries, when diets were limited by seasonal scarcity and lack of nutritional understanding, reaching 50 was considered remarkable. Today, guided by the wisdom of these centenarian cultures and supported by modern nutritional science, we can aspire to live not just longer, but healthier lives well into our later years.

The brain-nourishing aspects of these dietary traditions deserve special attention. The omega-3 rich fish consumption of both regions, combined with abundant polyphenols from olive oil, green tea, and colorful vegetables, provides powerful protection against cognitive decline. These neuroprotective elements, when paired with mindful eating practices and proper portion control, create an optimal environment for brain health - a crucial factor in preventing age-related cognitive conditions.

Perhaps most significantly, we've learned that longevity through diet isn't about deprivation or strict rules, but rather about embracing a rich tapestry of wholesome foods and mindful practices. The synthesis of Mediterranean and Japanese dietary wisdom offers us a flexible, enjoyable approach to eating that can be adapted to modern life while maintaining its core benefits.

As we move forward, let's remember that these dietary traditions are more than just meal plans - they're comprehensive approaches to nourishing both body and mind. By incorporating their principles into our daily lives, we can work toward achieving the remarkable longevity seen in the world's Blue Zones while enjoying the journey of discovering new flavors and traditions.

The path to longevity through diet is not about dramatic changes or extreme measures, but rather about making small, sustainable shifts in how we approach food and eating. Whether it's incorporating more plant-based foods, embracing fermented products, or practicing mindful eating, each step we take brings us closer to the wisdom that has sustained centenarians for generations.

As we close this chapter, remember that the power to influence your longevity through diet lies within your daily choices. The combined wisdom of Mediterranean and Japanese traditions, validated by modern science, provides us with a clear roadmap for eating our way to a longer, healthier life. Let this knowledge guide you as you create your own longevity-promoting dietary practices, always remembering that the best diet is one that you can maintain joyfully for a lifetime.

CHAPTER 4

Brain Longentity:

Ancient Practices and Modern Neuroscience for Cognitive Vitality

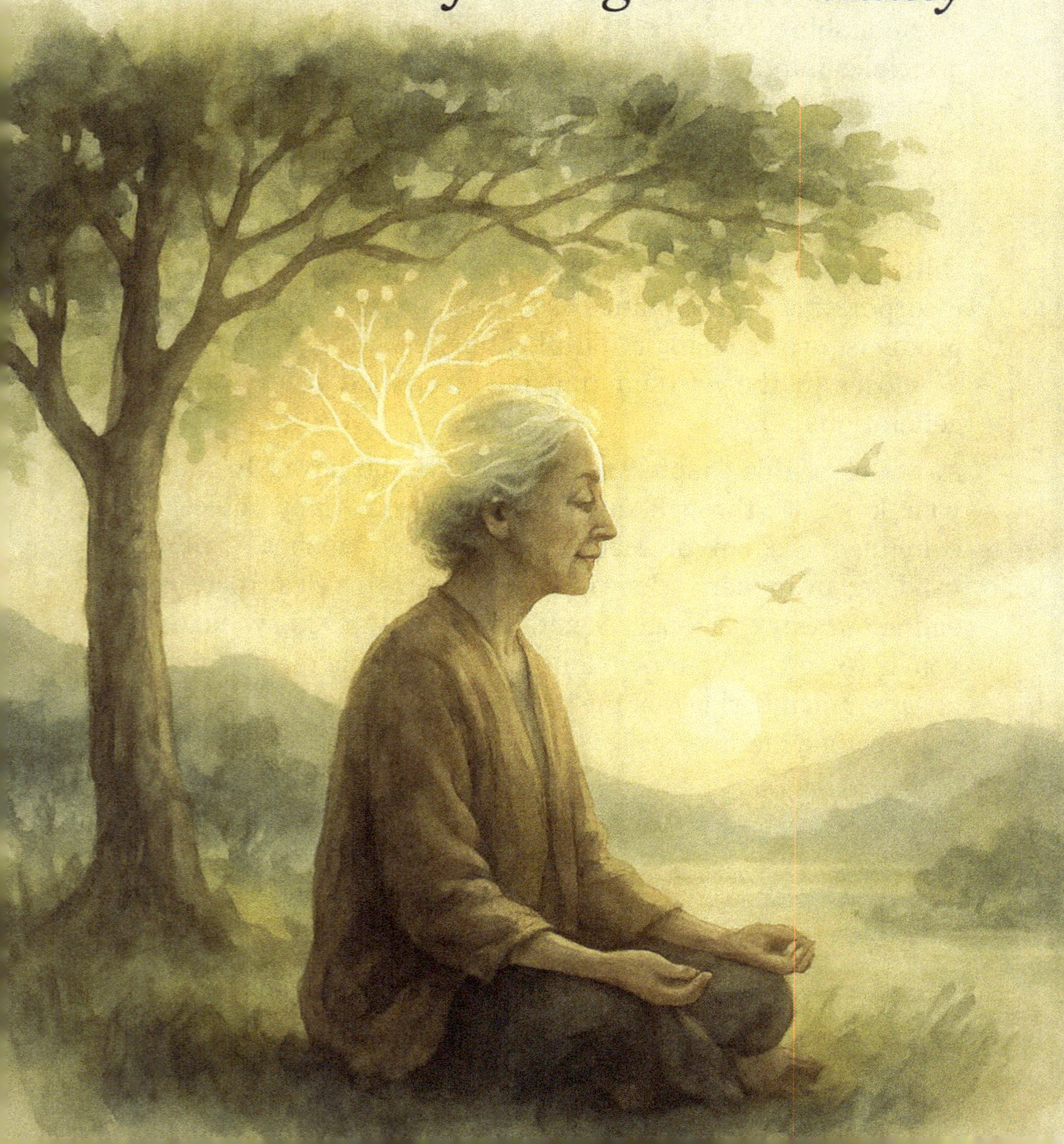

The human brain, with its remarkable capacity for adaptation and renewal, holds secrets that both ancient wisdom traditions and modern neuroscience are only beginning to unlock. While our ancestors may not have understood the intricate neural networks and biochemical processes, we now study, they developed powerful practices for maintaining cognitive vitality that modern research is validating and explaining at the molecular level. As we explore the intricate relationship between traditional brain-health practices and modern neuroscience, we uncover a fascinating tapestry of wisdom that spans generations and cultures. The brain's remarkable plasticity - its ability to form new neural connections throughout life - provides the foundation for both ancient cognitive preservation techniques and cutting-edge research in neuroscience.

In traditional societies, elders were revered not just for their wisdom, but for their ability to maintain sharp cognitive function well into their later years. These cultures developed sophisticated practices for preserving mental acuity, from specific meditation techniques to carefully crafted dietary protocols. What's particularly intriguing is how modern research continues to validate many of these ancestral approaches to brain health.

Consider the traditional practice of mindful eating in Japanese culture, where meals are consumed slowly and with full attention. Current neuroscience research has shown that this practice not only aids digestion but also strengthens neural pathways associated with attention and emotional regulation. Similarly, the ancient Indian practice of combining physical movement with memorization of verses has been shown to enhance both memory formation and retention.

Meet Tara, a remarkable cognitive neuroscientist who has experienced her own transformative journey with brain health. At age 45, after years of intense academic work that left her feeling mentally exhausted, she discovered that her grandmother's traditional practices for maintaining mental clarity aligned surprisingly well with her laboratory research. Intrigued by this connection, Aria began incorporating her grandmother's daily rituals - including specific breathing exercises, particular herbal teas, and memory games passed down through generations - alongside her modern understanding of neuroscience. She documented how these practices influenced various aspects of cognitive function, from attention span to memory retention. The most fascinating aspect was how her grandmother's insistence on regular social gatherings and storytelling perfectly matched current research on social engagement and cognitive preservation. After three years of combining these ancient practices with modern techniques, Aria not only experienced improved mental clarity and memory but also developed a groundbreaking program that helped others maintain their cognitive vitality. Her story beautifully illustrates how ancient wisdom and modern science can work together to support brain health, showing that our ancestors' intuitive understanding of cognitive maintenance often parallels contemporary scientific discoveries.

As we delve deeper into this chapter, we'll explore specific techniques that bridge the gap between traditional wisdom and modern neuroscience. We'll examine how practices like meditation physically alter brain structure, how certain traditional foods contain compounds now proven to support neuroplasticity, and how ancient memory techniques align with our current understanding of cognitive enhancement. Most importantly, we'll learn how to integrate these timeless practices into our modern lives in ways that are both practical and effective.

Meditation and Mindfulness: Traditional Practices Through a Neuroscientific Lens

The intersection of ancient meditation practices and modern neuroscience reveals fascinating insights into how contemplative traditions can enhance cognitive longevity. While our ancestors developed these practices through careful observation and generational wisdom, today's advanced imaging and research techniques allow us to understand the profound neurobiological effects of meditation on the aging brain.

Research conducted at Harvard Medical School by Dr. Sara Lazar has demonstrated that long-term meditators show increased cortical thickness in brain regions associated with attention and sensory processing. These areas are typically thin with age, but regular meditation appears to help preserve their structure and function. This scientific validation of ancient practices is particularly significant when we consider that our ancestors rarely lived beyond 40 years, while today we regularly see individuals maintaining sharp cognitive function well into their 80s and beyond.

The traditional practice of focused attention meditation, which involves concentrating on a single object like the breath, has been shown to enhance activity in the prefrontal cortex - an area crucial for executive function and working memory. Studies at the University of Wisconsin-Madison's Center for Healthy Minds have documented how this type of meditation can actually increase the density of gray matter in brain regions essential for learning, memory, and emotional regulation.

Particularly compelling is the research on mindfulness meditation's effect on cellular aging. Studies have revealed that regular meditation practice increases telomerase activity, an enzyme that protects DNA from age-related damage. This finding provides a potential biological mechanism for how ancient contemplative practices might contribute to longevity at the cellular level.

In Okinawa, where an unusually high percentage of the population lives past 100 years, daily mindfulness practices are seamlessly integrated into community life[27] [11]. These centenarians often engage in regular meditation as part of their daily routines, combining it with social interaction and purposeful activity - a holistic approach that modern neuroscience now confirms as beneficial for brain health.

The traditional Buddhist practice of Vipassana meditation, which emphasizes non-judgmental awareness of present-moment experience, has been shown through functional MRI studies to strengthen neural networks associated with attention and emotional regulation. This enhanced neural connectivity may help explain why long-term practitioners often maintain better cognitive function as they age.

Modern research has also validated the traditional wisdom of combining movement with meditation. Practices like walking meditation and tai chi have been shown to stimulate the production of brain-derived neurotrophic factor (BDNF), a protein that supports the survival of existing neurons and encourages the growth of new ones. This finding helps explain why contemplative movement practices have been associated with better cognitive outcomes in aging populations.

Perhaps most remarkably, studies have shown that even short periods of regular meditation can lead to measurable changes in brain structure and function. Research at UCLA found that long-term meditators had better-preserved brains than non-meditators as they aged, with more gray matter volume throughout the brain. These findings suggest that incorporating meditation into daily life could be one of the most effective strategies for maintaining cognitive vitality as we age.

Science is clear: traditional meditation practices offer powerful tools for protecting and enhancing brain health throughout life. By combining these ancient techniques with our modern understanding of neuroscience, we can develop more effective strategies for maintaining cognitive function well into our later years. The key lies not in choosing between traditional wisdom and modern science, but in understanding how they complement and validate each other, offering a more complete picture of how to support brain health and longevity[18].

Neuroprotective Nutrients: Ancient Diets and Brain-Boosting Foods

Throughout human history, our ancestors developed sophisticated dietary practices that modern science is now validating as powerful tools for brain health and longevity. While early humans rarely lived beyond their fourth decade due to harsh environmental conditions, limited medical knowledge, and inadequate nutrition, their dietary wisdom laid the groundwork for our understanding of neuroprotective nutrients. Today, as we regularly live into our 80s and beyond, these ancient nutritional practices have become even more relevant for maintaining cognitive vitality throughout our extended lifespans.

The Mediterranean diet, with its emphasis on olive oil, nuts, whole grains, and fish, has emerged as a powerful blueprint for brain health. Research has shown that its rich combination of omega-3 fatty acids, polyphenols, and antioxidants supports neuronal membrane integrity and reduces inflammation - key factors in preventing cognitive decline[28]. This traditional eating pattern, developed over millennia in the Mediterranean basin, provides compelling evidence for how ancestral wisdom can align with modern neuroscience.

In Okinawa, where an extraordinary number of residents live past 100 years with remarkable cognitive clarity, the traditional diet centers around sweet potatoes, tofu, seaweed, and fish. This nutrient-dense combination provides a wealth of flavonoids, carotenoids, and omega-3s that modern research has linked to enhanced brain function and reduced risk of neurodegenerative diseases[28]. The Okinawan example demonstrates how specific dietary patterns can contribute to both longevity and cognitive preservation.

Modern neuroscience has identified several key neuroprotective nutrients that were inadvertently abundant in traditional diets. Omega-3 fatty acids, found in fatty fish and walnuts, support synaptic plasticity and reduce inflammation[30]. Polyphenols and flavonoids, present in berries, tea, and cocoa, boost cerebral blood flow and may help clear harmful proteins from the brain[28]. Curcumin, the active compound in turmeric, has been shown to inhibit neuroinflammation and reduce oxidative stress[28].

B vitamins, particularly B6, B9, and B12, play crucial roles in homocysteine metabolism and neurotransmitter synthesis. Traditional diets rich in organ meats, legumes, and leafy greens naturally provided these essential nutrients. Their deficiency has been linked to cognitive impairment and increased risk of Alzheimer's disease, highlighting the importance of maintaining adequate levels through diet or supplementation when necessary.

The synergistic effects of combining these brain-boosting foods are particularly noteworthy. Traditional Asian diets, for instance, typically combine fish (omega-3s) with green tea (EGCG) and turmeric (curcumin), creating a powerful neuroprotective effect that exceeds the benefits of any single component[28]. This holistic approach to nutrition reflects an intuitive understanding of food combinations that modern research continues to validate.

To optimize brain health in our modern context, we can learn from these traditional dietary patterns while incorporating current scientific insights. A brain-healthy diet should emphasize plant-based foods rich in antioxidants, include regular consumption of fatty fish, incorporate fermented foods for gut health, and maintain adequate levels of essential nutrients through varied food sources.

Practical steps for implementing these principles include consuming fatty fish at least twice weekly, incorporating a variety of colorful fruits and vegetables daily, using herbs and spices liberally (particularly turmeric with black pepper), and choosing whole grains over refined carbohydrates. Additionally, maintaining adequate hydration and limiting processed foods helps create an optimal environment for brain health.

The evidence suggests that adopting these dietary practices early and maintaining them throughout life provides the greatest benefit for cognitive longevity. However, research also indicates that it's never too late to start - even modest dietary improvements in later life can support brain health and potentially slow cognitive decline[28].

While genetics play a role in extreme longevity, with studies suggesting about 40% genetic influence in centenarians[29][30], dietary choices remain a powerful tool for supporting cognitive health throughout life. By combining ancient dietary wisdom with modern nutritional science, we can create eating patterns that support not just longer lives, but sharper, more vibrant cognitive function well into our later years.

Cognitive Exercise: Traditional Memory Techniques and Modern Brain Training

Throughout human history, memory techniques have been vital tools for preserving knowledge and wisdom across generations. In ancient times, when written records were scarce and lifespans rarely exceeded 40 years, these cognitive practices were essential for cultural survival. Today, as we regularly live into our 80s and beyond, these traditional memory techniques have taken on new significance in our quest for cognitive longevity.

The ancient Greeks developed one of the most powerful memory systems known as the Method of Loci, where information is visualized within specific spatial locations. This technique, famously used by Roman orator Cicero, remains remarkably effective today. Modern neuroscience has validated its efficacy, showing that spatial memory engages multiple brain regions, creating robust neural networks that support cognitive resilience.

In traditional societies, memory techniques were deeply integrated into daily life. The Yoruba oral poets of West Africa, for instance, developed intricate rhythmic recitation methods to preserve vast genealogies, while Aboriginal Australians encoded navigational and historical information through Songlines. These practices didn't just preserve information - they actively exercised the brain in ways that modern neuroscience now recognizes as beneficial for cognitive health.

Dr. Michael Merzenich, a leading neuroscientist, emphasizes that "The brain is plastic and continually shaped by experience—cognitive exercise is as essential to brain health as physical exercise is to body health." This understanding has led to the development of modern brain training programs that aim to harness this neuroplasticity. However, research suggests that the most effective approach combines traditional memory techniques with contemporary cognitive training.

The ACTIVE Study (Advanced Cognitive Training for Independent and Vital Elderly) has demonstrated that older adults who engage in structured cognitive training can maintain improved reasoning and processing speed for up to ten years[18]. This research validates what traditional cultures inherently understood - regular mental exercise is crucial for maintaining cognitive vitality.

Practical implementation of cognitive exercise should include both traditional and modern approaches. Key strategies include:

- Regular practice of visualization and association techniques

- Engagement with novel, complex activities like learning new languages
- Participation in group-based memory games and discussions
- Integration of traditional mnemonic practices with digital brain training platforms

The synergy between ancient wisdom and modern science becomes particularly evident when examining the mechanisms of memory enhancement. Traditional techniques like chunking (grouping information into meaningful units) and peg systems (linking items to pre-memorized lists) align perfectly with our current understanding of how the brain processes and stores information.

Dr. Anders Ericsson, an expert on expertise and memory, notes that "What sets expert performers apart is not experience per se, but the amount of deliberate practice—purposeful and systematic cognitive exercise." This insight applies equally to maintaining cognitive health as we age. The key is not just engaging in mental activities, but ensuring they are sufficiently challenging and systematically practiced.

Modern brain training programs have emerged as powerful tools for cognitive enhancement, offering structured activities that target specific cognitive domains. While these digital platforms provide immediate feedback and adaptive difficulty levels, research indicates they are most effective when combined with traditional memory techniques and social engagement.

The evidence suggests that cognitive exercise is most beneficial when integrated into a holistic approach to brain health. This includes maintaining a neuroprotective diet, engaging in regular physical activity, ensuring adequate sleep, and fostering strong social connections. The combination of these factors creates an optimal environment for cognitive preservation and enhancement.

As we continue to push the boundaries of human longevity, the importance of maintaining cognitive vitality becomes increasingly crucial. By combining the wisdom of traditional memory techniques with insights from modern neuroscience, we can develop more effective strategies for preserving and enhancing cognitive function throughout our extended lifespans. The key lies not in choosing between old and new approaches, but in understanding how they complement each other to support optimal brain health.

Social Engagement and Brain Health: Community Practices Across Cultures

Throughout human history, social bonds have been crucial not just for survival but for maintaining cognitive vitality. In earlier times, when life expectancy rarely exceeded 40 years due to harsh conditions, infectious diseases, and limited medical knowledge, communities relied on social structures to preserve knowledge and support collective survival. Today, as we regularly live into our 80s and beyond, research reveals that these traditional social practices hold profound implications for brain health and longevity.

Modern neuroscience has validated what many traditional cultures inherently understood - that regular social engagement significantly reduces the risk of cognitive decline. Studies show that individuals with strong social connections have a 30-50% lower risk of developing dementia, with this protective effect linked to increased cognitive reserve and improved cerebrovascular health[31]. This finding is particularly significant as we consider how to maintain brain vitality throughout our extended modern lifespans.

Across different cultures, we find remarkable examples of social practices that promote cognitive health. In Okinawa, Japan, the traditional "moai" system - mutual support groups that meet regularly for social, financial, and emotional support - has been associated with exceptional mental clarity among their centenarian population. These groups provide not just companionship but also purposeful engagement that challenges the brain in multiple ways.

In Mediterranean societies, particularly in Sardinia, community practices center around regular communal meals, religious gatherings, and neighborhood social clubs. These activities create environments rich in social interaction, emotional support, and cognitive stimulation. Advanced brain imaging studies reveal that older adults who participate in such regular social activities show more robust gray matter integrity in regions relevant to dementia prevention[32].

The mechanisms through which social engagement supports brain health are multiple and interconnected. Regular social interaction reduces chronic stress, which is known to damage critical brain regions like the hippocampus and prefrontal cortex[31]. Additionally, social activities stimulate neuroplasticity - the brain's ability to form new neural connections throughout life. The emotional support provided through strong social bonds creates psychological resilience, which further protects against cognitive decline[33].

Modern research has identified specific types of social engagement that appear particularly beneficial for brain health. Group activities such as board games, movie outings, travel, educational classes, and religious services have been linked to higher scores in brain health and microstructural integrity[32]. Importantly, it's not just the quantity but the quality of social connections that matters - meaningful friendships and supportive relationships appear to have the strongest protective effects[33].

In institutional settings like long-term care facilities, the importance of social engagement becomes even more critical. While these environments can sometimes limit social opportunities, efforts to expand social networks through structured group activities and facilitation of meaningful connections can help counteract isolation and support cognitive health[33]. This understanding has led to innovations in care facility design and programming that prioritize social interaction.

Dr. Cynthia Felix from the University of Pittsburgh Graduate School of Public Health suggests that "Prescribing socialization could benefit older adults in warding off dementia, much the way prescribing physical activity can help to prevent diabetes or heart disease."[32] This medical perspective on social engagement represents a significant shift in how we approach brain health and cognitive preservation.

To optimize brain health in our modern context, it's essential to create regular opportunities for meaningful social interaction. This might include joining community groups, participating in volunteer activities, engaging in group exercise classes, or simply maintaining regular contact with friends and family. The key is consistency and genuine engagement rather than passive social presence.

While social participation is clearly linked to reduced dementia risk, researchers note that healthier brains may enable greater social engagement, creating a positive feedback loop[32,33]. This understanding emphasizes the importance of establishing strong social connections early in life and maintaining them throughout our extended lifespans.

As we continue to push the boundaries of human longevity, the role of social engagement in maintaining cognitive vitality becomes increasingly crucial. By combining traditional community practices with modern understanding of brain health, we can create social environments that support not just longer lives, but sharper, more vibrant cognitive function well into our later years[31,32,33,34].

Sleep Optimization: Traditional Wisdom and Modern Sleep Science

Throughout human history, sleep has been recognized as a cornerstone of health and longevity. In earlier times, when life expectancy rarely exceeded 40 years due to infectious diseases, harsh living conditions, and limited medical knowledge, traditional cultures developed sophisticated practices for optimizing sleep quality. Today, as we regularly live into our 80s and beyond, these ancient sleep wisdom traditions have taken on new significance, particularly in their ability to support cognitive health and longevity.

Modern neuroscience has validated what many traditional societies inherently understood - that quality sleep is essential for brain health and cognitive preservation. Research shows that during sleep, the brain undergoes crucial maintenance processes, including the clearance of harmful proteins associated with neurodegenerative diseases. This understanding adds new weight to traditional practices that prioritized proper sleep hygiene.

Across different cultures, we find remarkable similarities in traditional sleep optimization practices. Evening relaxation rituals, including gentle movement and warm baths 60-90 minutes before bedtime, were common practices that modern science now confirms can trigger the "temperature-drop effect" necessary for quality sleep[35]. As noted in traditional Chinese medicine, "Eating too much at dinner shortens your lifespan by a day,"[38] - wisdom that aligns with contemporary research on the relationship between meal timing and sleep quality.

The synchronization of sleep patterns with natural light was a fundamental aspect of traditional sleep practices. Before artificial lighting disrupted our natural rhythms, communities naturally aligned their sleep-wake cycles with the sun's patterns[36]. This practice, we now know, optimizes the production of melatonin, our primary sleep hormone, and supports the body's circadian rhythm - a crucial factor in both sleep quality and cognitive health[35][36].

Modern research has identified specific mechanisms through which traditional sleep practices support brain health. Controlled breathing techniques, such as box breathing and extended exhalation, have been shown to calm the nervous system and reduce cortisol levels, preparing the body and mind for restorative sleep[35] [36]. Similarly, traditional practices of maintaining cool sleeping environments (65-68°F / 18-20°C) and using natural aromatherapy align with our current understanding of optimal sleep conditions[35].

The timing of meals, particularly in relation to sleep, has emerged as a critical factor in both sleep quality and longevity. Traditional wisdom advocating for light, early dinners is supported by modern research showing that eating the last meal 3-4 hours before bedtime supports metabolic health, reduces inflammation, and aligns with the body's natural detoxification processes[37] [38]. This practice becomes increasingly important as we aim to maintain cognitive vitality throughout our extended modern lifespans.

Environmental modifications play a crucial role in sleep optimization. While our ancestors naturally reduced light exposure after sunset, today we must consciously manage our exposure to artificial light, particularly blue light from electronic devices. Wearing blue light-blocking glasses or reducing screen exposure before bed helps prevent circadian disruption and supports natural sleep patterns[37].

The integration of traditional sleep wisdom with modern science offers powerful strategies for optimizing brain health and longevity. Key practices include adopting evening wind-down rituals, maintaining consistent sleep-wake cycles aligned with natural light patterns, practicing proper breathing techniques, and creating optimal sleeping environments. These practices not only support immediate sleep quality but also contribute to long-term cognitive preservation.

As Dr. James Liu, a prominent sleep researcher, notes, "When we combine traditional wisdom with modern understanding of sleep physiology, we create powerful rituals that honor our biological need for proper transitions."[35] This synthesis of ancient wisdom and contemporary science provides a comprehensive approach to sleep optimization that supports both immediate well-being and long-term cognitive vitality.

By understanding and implementing these time-tested sleep practices, while adapting them to our modern context, we can create sleep routines that support optimal brain health throughout our extended lifespans. The key lies not in choosing between traditional wisdom and modern science, but in understanding how they complement each other to support restful, restorative sleep - a fundamental pillar of cognitive longevity.As we conclude our exploration of brain longevity and cognitive vitality, it's remarkable to reflect on how far human understanding of brain health has evolved. In earlier times, when life expectancy rarely exceeded 40 years due to infectious diseases, harsh living conditions, and limited medical knowledge, maintaining cognitive function into advanced age wasn't a primary concern. Today, as we regularly live into our 80s and beyond, the intersection of ancient wisdom and modern neuroscience offers unprecedented opportunities for preserving and enhancing our cognitive capabilities.

Throughout this chapter, we've discovered how traditional practices for maintaining mental acuity align remarkably well with current scientific understanding. From the mindfulness techniques that physically alter brain structure to the neuroprotective nutrients found in traditional diets, we've seen how ancestral wisdom often anticipated what modern research would later confirm. The story of Tara, the cognitive neuroscientist who combined her grandmother's traditional practices with contemporary research, illustrates the powerful potential of bridging these two worlds.

Key insights from our exploration reveal several fundamental principles for maintaining cognitive vitality:

- Regular meditation and mindfulness practices physically alter brain structure and enhance neural connectivity

- A diet rich in traditional neuroprotective nutrients supports brain health and reduces inflammation

- Traditional memory techniques, when combined with modern cognitive training, create robust neural networks
- Strong social connections significantly reduce the risk of cognitive decline
- Quality sleep, guided by both ancient wisdom and modern science, is essential for brain maintenance

As we move forward in our longevity journey, it's crucial to remember that cognitive health isn't just about preventing decline - it's about optimizing our brain's remarkable potential throughout life. The practices we've explored support not just longer lives, but sharper, more vibrant cognitive function well into our later years.

By combining traditional wisdom with modern scientific understanding, we can create powerful strategies for maintaining cognitive vitality. Whether it's incorporating mindfulness practices into daily routines, adopting brain-healthy dietary habits, or maintaining strong social connections, each step we take supports our brain's remarkable capacity for adaptation and renewal.

Remember, it's never too early - or too late - to begin implementing these practices. The brain's plasticity means that positive changes can occur at any age, though the benefits are greatest when healthy habits are established early and maintained consistently. As we continue to push the boundaries of human longevity, maintaining cognitive vitality becomes increasingly crucial for enjoying our extended lifespans to the fullest.

In the next chapter, we'll explore how traditional food preservation techniques not only extended our ancestors' food supply but also enhanced their nutritional intake in ways that modern science is only beginning to understand. The fascinating world of fermentation awaits, offering another powerful tool in our quest for optimal health and longevity.

CHAPTER 5

The Fermentation Factor:
Reviving Ancient Techniques for Modern Gut Health

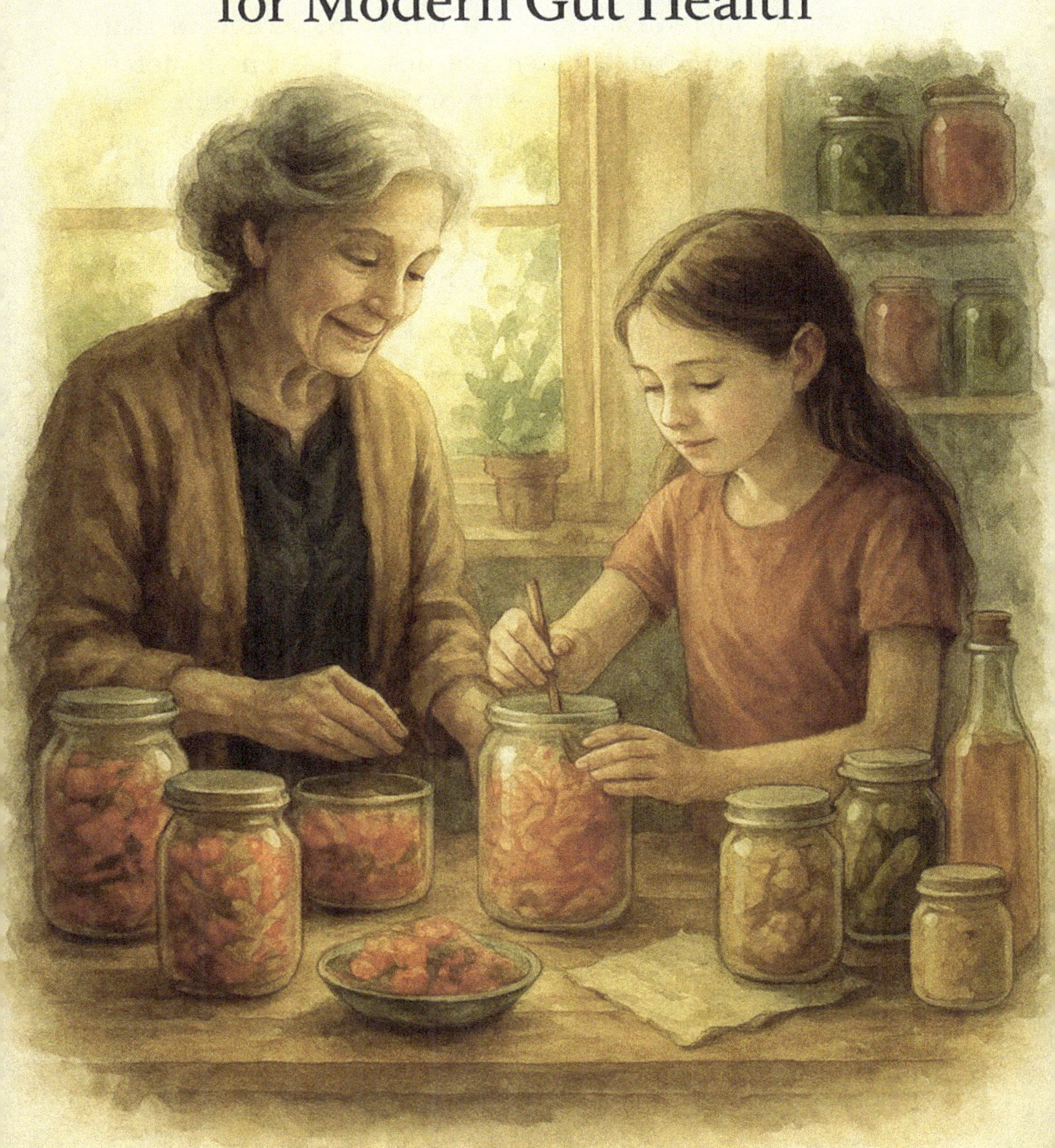

Across the misty mountains of Korea and the verdant valleys of the Caucasus, ancient communities discovered a transformative alchemy in the art of fermentation, turning simple ingredients into nutritional powerhouses that could sustain life through harsh seasons. This time-honored practice, which began as a necessity for food preservation, has emerged as a cornerstone of gut health and longevity in our modern understanding of nutrition. In ancient food preservation techniques lies a profound connection to human health that modern science is only beginning to fully comprehend. From the kimchi pots buried in Korean courtyards to the sourdough cultures passed down through generations in European bakeries, these traditional methods have sustained communities for millennia while unknowingly cultivating beneficial microorganisms that we now know are crucial for human health.

The art of fermentation represents one of humanity's earliest forms of food technology, born from necessity but perfected through careful observation and cultural wisdom. This transformative process not only preserved food for lean times but enhanced its nutritional value in ways our ancestors understood intuitively, if not scientifically. What they observed through generations of practice, we can now explain through the lens of microbiology - how beneficial bacteria transform simple ingredients into probiotic-rich foods that support our gut microbiome and overall health.

During my research into traditional food preservation methods, I became familiar with Blake, a former chef turned fermentation enthusiast who discovered these ancient practices while seeking solutions for his own health challenges. At age forty, struggling with chronic digestive issues and inflammation, Blake began exploring traditional fermentation techniques from various cultures. He started with simple sauerkraut, following methods passed down through generations of Eastern European families, then expanded his repertoire to include Korean kimchi, Japanese miso, and Caucasian milk kefir. The transformation in his health was remarkable - his digestive issues resolved, his energy levels soared, and his inflammatory markers decreased significantly. What began as a personal health journey evolved into a passion for teaching others. Blake now runs workshops teaching traditional fermentation techniques adapted for modern kitchens, helping people reconnect with these ancient practices of food preservation and health promotion. His story particularly resonated with me because it demonstrated how ancient wisdom could provide solutions to modern health challenges, bridging the gap between traditional food preservation and contemporary wellness needs.

In this chapter, we'll explore how these time-honored practices of fermentation and food preservation not only kept our ancestors alive through harsh seasons but may hold the key to addressing many modern health challenges. We'll examine the science behind these traditional methods and discover practical ways to incorporate them into our contemporary lifestyles. By understanding both the cultural wisdom and scientific principles of fermentation, we can harness this ancient art to support our health and longevity in the modern world.

Global Fermentation Traditions: From Kimchi to Kefir

Across the world's most vibrant centenarian communities, one common thread emerges consistently - the daily consumption of traditionally fermented foods[40]. From the mountainous regions of the Caucasus to the coastal villages of Korea, these time-tested preservation techniques have not only sustained communities through harsh seasons but have also contributed significantly to their remarkable longevity. Modern science now validates what these cultures have known intuitively for generations - fermented foods play a crucial role in maintaining gut health, supporting immune function, and potentially even protecting cognitive health as we age[42][43].

In Korea, the art of kimchi-making represents more than just food preservation; it embodies a cultural legacy of health and longevity. Traditional kimchi contains napa cabbage, radish, chili, garlic, and ginger, fermented through a carefully monitored process that produces beneficial probiotics[39]. Research has linked regular kimchi consumption to lower cholesterol levels, reduced insulin resistance, and improved gut health[39][40][41]. The practice of kimjang - the communal preparation of kimchi - showcases how these traditional preservation methods fostered both physical health and social bonds, two critical factors in longevity.

Moving westward to the Caucasus Mountains, we find the birthplace of kefir, a fermented dairy drink that has been central to the exceptional longevity of local populations for centuries[41]. Made by fermenting milk with kefir grains - a complex symbiotic mix of bacteria and yeast - this probiotic-rich beverage offers unique health benefits. Scientific studies have shown that kefir's probiotics may reduce inflammation, enhance immunity, and improve glucose metabolism[39][41]. The traditional practice of sharing kefir grains between families created not just a sustainable food system but also strengthened community bonds, another vital factor in longevity.

In Japan, the daily consumption of miso, a fermented soybean paste, has been linked to better digestive health and cardiovascular function[39]. Traditional miso-making involves a lengthy fermentation process using koji mold, resulting in a protein-rich condiment packed with beneficial compounds. Research has shown that regular miso consumption may contribute to the remarkably low rates of certain chronic diseases in traditional Japanese populations.

The science behind these traditional practices reveals why fermented foods have such profound health impacts. During fermentation, beneficial microorganisms break down hard-to-digest compounds, create new nutrients, and produce postbiotics that support our gut microbiome[39]. This enhanced nutritional profile, combined with the live beneficial bacteria, helps explain why communities with regular fermented food consumption often display better health outcomes and increased longevity[40][41][43].

Modern research has revealed another fascinating aspect of fermented foods - their potential impact on brain health. The gut-brain axis, a bidirectional communication system between our digestive tract and nervous system, appears to be positively influenced by the regular consumption of fermented foods[40][41]. Studies suggest that the probiotics and bioactive compounds in these traditional foods may help reduce inflammation and oxidative stress, two factors implicated in cognitive decline.

For those seeking to incorporate these traditional wisdom practices into modern life, it's essential to understand that not all fermented products offer equal benefits. Traditional, naturally fermented foods containing live cultures provide the most significant health advantages[42]. Mass-produced versions often lack the microbial diversity and beneficial compounds found in traditionally prepared ferments. When selecting fermented foods, look for those made using traditional methods and containing live, active cultures[42].

The global tradition of fermentation reminds us that some of the most powerful tools for health and longevity have been hiding in plain sight, preserved in the cultural practices of the world's longest-living populations[40]. By understanding and adopting these time-tested methods while honoring their traditional preparation techniques, we can harness their benefits for modern health and longevity[43].

The Microbiome Connection: How Fermented Foods Support Gut Health

The intricate relationship between fermented foods and our gut microbiome represents one of the most fascinating discoveries in modern longevity research, bridging ancient wisdom with cutting-edge science. Our ancestors, who typically lived shorter lives due to various environmental and health challenges, unknowingly cultivated powerful allies in their quest for survival through the practice of fermentation. Today, we understand that these traditional food preservation techniques not only kept our forebears alive through lean times but also nourished the complex ecosystem of microorganisms in their digestive systems - a key factor in modern longevity[44][46].

The human gut houses trillions of microorganisms, collectively known as the microbiome, which plays a crucial role in everything from digestion to immune function and even brain health[44][45][46]. Dr. Suzanne Devkota of Cedars-Sinai emphasizes that "most fermented foods contain probiotics, which are the good bacteria that support our gut health."[44] This understanding helps explain why communities with traditional fermented foods in their daily diets often display remarkable longevity and cognitive vitality well into their later years[46].

A groundbreaking Stanford clinical trial demonstrated the profound impact of fermented foods on our internal ecosystem. Participants who consumed fermented foods daily for ten weeks showed increased microbial diversity and reduced inflammatory markers in their bodies[45]. Dr. Justin Sonnenburg, associate professor at Stanford, noted this study "provides one of the first examples of how a simple change in diet can reproducibly remodel the microbiota across a cohort of healthy adults."[45]

The microbiome's influence extends beyond digestion to impact our brain health significantly. Through the gut-brain axis, these beneficial microorganisms communicate with our nervous system, potentially influencing cognitive function and emotional well-being[44] [46]. Regular consumption of fermented foods has been linked to reduced inflammation throughout the body, including the brain, which may help protect against age-related cognitive decline[44] [45].

Fermented foods support our microbiome through multiple mechanisms. They provide live beneficial bacteria that can populate the gut, crowding out harmful pathogens[44] [46]. Even when these microbes are inactive, their fermentation produces valuable compounds called postbiotics that interact with our immune system and strengthen the gut barrier[44]. These foods also increase the bioavailability of essential nutrients, including B vitamins and vitamin K, which are crucial for brain health and longevity[44].

Dr. David S. Ludwig of Harvard T.H. Chan School of Public Health emphasizes that "research today is revealing the importance of a diverse and healthy intestinal microbiome because it plays a role in fine-tuning the immune system and wards off damaging inflammation inside the body."[46] This inflammation reduction is particularly significant as chronic inflammation has been identified as a major factor in accelerated aging and cognitive decline[44] [45].

The connection between fermented foods and longevity becomes even more apparent when we examine traditional diets in regions known for their centenarian populations. In these areas, fermented foods like miso, kimchi, and yogurt are dietary staples, consumed daily as part of a balanced, whole-food diet. Population studies consistently link their regular consumption to better digestive health and lower incidence of inflammatory disorders[46].

However, it's important to note that not all fermented products offer equal benefits. Mass-produced versions often lack the microbial diversity and beneficial compounds found in traditionally prepared ferments[44]. When selecting fermented foods, look for those made using traditional methods and containing live, active cultures. This attention to quality ensures you're getting the full spectrum of microbiome-supporting benefits that have contributed to human health and longevity for generations[44].

By understanding and harnessing the power of fermented foods, we can actively support our gut microbiome, potentially extending both our lifespan and our healthspan[44][46]. This ancient practice, validated by modern science, offers a practical strategy for maintaining cognitive vitality and overall health as we age - a testament to the enduring wisdom of traditional food preservation methods[44][45][46].

Traditional Preservation Techniques and Their Modern Applications

Long before the advent of modern refrigeration and food science, our ancestors developed ingenious methods for preserving food that not only ensured survival through lean times but also inadvertently created powerful allies for human health and longevity. These traditional preservation techniques - from sun-drying and smoking to fermentation and salting - emerged as early as 12,000 BC in the Middle East[47][49], marking humanity's first steps toward food security and extended lifespans.

In ancient Mesopotamia and Rome, salt became so precious for its preservation properties that it served as currency[47], highlighting the critical role of food preservation in human civilization. The ability to preserve food through various methods meant communities could maintain nutritional stability year-round, gradually contributing to increased life expectancy. Traditional preservation techniques didn't just prevent spoilage; they often enhanced the nutritional value of foods in ways we're only now beginning to fully understand through modern science.

Drying, one of the oldest preservation methods, demonstrates the elegant simplicity of traditional techniques. By removing moisture through exposure to sun, wind, or controlled heat, our ancestors created an environment inhospitable to microbial growth while concentrating nutrients in foods. European monks took this practice further by building specialized "still houses" for drying in regions with limited sunlight[47], showing how these techniques evolved to meet local environmental challenges.

Smoking, which naturally evolved from drying practices, added another dimension to food preservation. The process not only dehydrates food but also imparts antimicrobial compounds such as phenols, creating a dual preservation effect[47]. This technique, still valued today, showcases how traditional methods often employed multiple mechanisms to ensure food safety and longevity.

Perhaps most fascinating is how these ancient preservation techniques often enhanced rather than merely maintained nutritional value. Fermentation, likely discovered by accident in early agricultural societies[48], transforms foods through beneficial microorganisms, increasing vitamin content (particularly B vitamins and vitamin K) and improving nutrient bioavailability[48]. Modern research validates what our ancestors knew intuitively - these preserved foods contributed significantly to their health and survival.

Today, these traditional preservation methods are experiencing a renaissance as we recognize their potential contributions to modern health challenges. The National Center for Home Food Preservation notes that fermentation not only preserves food but creates more nutritious products through microbial activity[48]. This understanding has led to a revival of traditional preservation techniques among health-conscious consumers seeking both practical and nutritional benefits[50].

The sustainability aspect of traditional preservation methods also resonates with modern concerns. These techniques typically require minimal technological intervention and are remarkably energy-efficient, offering valuable lessons for contemporary food systems. By preserving seasonal abundance through traditional methods, we can reduce food waste while maintaining nutritional quality - a practice that bridges ancient wisdom with modern needs.

For those seeking to incorporate these traditional preservation techniques into modern life, it's essential to understand both their historical context and scientific principles. While our ancestors may not have understood the molecular mechanisms behind these preservation methods, their careful observations and refined techniques created a legacy of food preservation that continues to offer insights into health and longevity. By combining this ancestral wisdom with modern understanding, we can harness these time-tested techniques for optimal health while honoring the ingenuity of traditional food preservation practices.

Nutrient Enhancement Through Fermentation

The ancient art of fermentation not only preserved food but also unlocked hidden nutritional treasures that our ancestors, who often lived shorter lives due to various health challenges, unknowingly harnessed for their survival. Modern science has revealed that this traditional preservation method actually enhances the nutrient content of foods in remarkable ways, potentially contributing to our increased longevity compared to earlier generations. Through the complex biochemical changes facilitated by beneficial microorganisms, fermentation transforms simple ingredients into nutritional powerhouses that support both gut and brain health[51][46].

One of the most fascinating aspects of fermentation is its ability to reduce anti-nutritional compounds while simultaneously increasing nutrient bioavailability. As Dr. David S. Ludwig from Harvard T.H. Chan School of Public Health notes, "Most societies throughout the world and throughout time have included fermented foods as part of their diet."[46] This universal practice has profound implications - during fermentation, microbial enzymes break down substances like tannins and phytates that typically bind minerals and limit their absorption. This process releases essential nutrients, including calcium, iron, and zinc, making them more accessible to our bodies[51][53].

The vitamin-enhancing properties of fermentation are particularly noteworthy. Beneficial bacteria involved in the fermentation process can actually synthesize new vitamins, including vital B vitamins and vitamin K. For instance, certain strains of Bacillus subtilis, found in traditional Japanese natto, produce significant amounts of vitamin K2, while other fermentation processes increase levels of riboflavin, thiamine, and even vitamin B12 - a nutrient typically absent in plant foods[51][46].

Perhaps most intriguing is fermentation's impact on brain health, a critical factor in modern longevity. The process creates bioactive compounds, including polyphenols and phenolic compounds with powerful antioxidant and anti-inflammatory properties[51][53]. These substances may help protect against cognitive decline by reducing oxidative stress and inflammation in the brain. Additionally, certain fermentation processes produce GABA (gamma-aminobutyric acid), a neurotransmitter linked to relaxation and reduced anxiety, potentially supporting both mental health and cognitive longevity[51].

The protein-enhancing effects of fermentation offer another layer of nutritional benefit. Through fermentation, proteins are partially broken down into more digestible forms, and the availability of essential amino acids increases[51]. This improved protein accessibility was particularly valuable for our ancestors, who often had limited access to animal proteins. Today, this benefit remains relevant for those following plant-based diets or seeking to optimize their protein intake for healthy aging[51].

Modern research has revealed that fermented foods contribute to longevity through multiple pathways. Beyond their enhanced nutrient profiles, these foods support a diverse gut microbiome, which is increasingly recognized as crucial for both physical and cognitive health. The probiotics in fermented foods help restore gut microbial balance, potentially reducing inflammation throughout the body and supporting immune function - key factors in healthy aging and disease prevention[52][46].

In Japan, where fermented foods like natto are dietary staples, populations demonstrate some of the world's highest rates of longevity. Epidemiological studies suggest that regular consumption of these traditional fermented foods contributes to cardiovascular health and bone density in aging populations[51][46]. This real-world evidence supports the scientific understanding of fermentation's role in enhancing nutrient availability and promoting overall health.

The transformation of simple ingredients into nutrient-rich foods through fermentation represents one of humanity's most significant nutritional achievements. While our ancestors may not have understood the molecular mechanisms at work, their traditional preservation practices created foods that not only sustained life but enhanced it. Today, as we face modern health challenges and seek ways to extend our healthspan, these ancient fermentation practices offer valuable lessons in nutrition and longevity[51][46][53].

Building a Modern Fermentation Practice: Safety and Methods

While our ancestors faced numerous challenges in food preservation that often contributed to shorter lifespans, modern fermentation practices combine their time-tested wisdom with scientific understanding to create safe, health-promoting foods. Dr. Robert W. Hutkins, a renowned microbiologist, emphasizes that "the safety of fermented foods relies on creating the right environmental conditions—acidity, salinity, and temperature—to favor beneficial microbes and exclude pathogens."[54] This understanding has transformed what was once a survival necessity into a powerful tool for promoting longevity and cognitive health.

The foundation of safe modern fermentation rests on what experts call the 3S Approach: Safety, Spoilage prevention, and Shelf-life management[54]. This systematic approach helps ensure that fermented foods not only preserve well but also maintain their brain-boosting potential through proper preparation and storage. The key to success lies in maintaining strict hygiene protocols while creating an environment that promotes beneficial bacterial growth while inhibiting harmful microorganisms.

To establish a safe fermentation practice, several critical elements must be in place. First, all equipment should be thoroughly cleaned with hot, soapy water and properly dried[54] [55]. While sterilization isn't mandatory, many practitioners prefer using boiling water or food-grade sanitizers for additional safety[55]. The choice of fermentation vessels is equally important - glass, food-grade plastics, or stainless steel are recommended, while reactive materials like aluminum or copper should be avoided as they can compromise both safety and nutritional value[55] [56].

Proper ingredient selection plays a crucial role in successful fermentation. Fresh, undamaged produce provides the best foundation for fermentation, as damaged or spoiled ingredients can introduce harmful microorganisms[54]. When working with dairy ferments, using pasteurized milk helps reduce pathogen risk while still allowing beneficial bacteria to thrive[54]. This attention to ingredient quality helps ensure that the final product will support rather than compromise our health.

Monitoring pH levels has emerged as a critical safety measure in modern fermentation. Using pH strips or digital meters, practitioners should aim for a final pH between 3.0 and 4.0 for vegetable ferments[55]. This acidic environment not only preserves food but also creates conditions that support cognitive health through the production of beneficial compounds and probiotics. A pH above 4.5 after five days may indicate unsafe fermentation and should prompt careful evaluation of the batch[55].

Temperature control represents another crucial aspect of safe fermentation. Most vegetable ferments perform best between 18–22°C (64–72°F)[54] [56]. This temperature range not only ensures food safety but also promotes the development of beneficial compounds that may support brain health and overall longevity. Once fermentation is complete, refrigeration helps maintain these benefits by slowing further microbial activity while extending shelf life.

Regular monitoring for signs of successful fermentation versus potential problems is essential. Healthy ferments should display a pleasantly sour or yeasty aroma, never rotten or putrid[54]. Visual inspection should reveal no fuzzy or black mold, and textures should remain firm rather than slimy[54] [55]. When in doubt, food safety experts unanimously recommend erring on the side of caution and discarding questionable batches[55].

The revival of traditional fermentation practices in the early 2000s demonstrated how combining ancient wisdom with modern safety protocols can create consistently safe, nutritious products[54] [56]. This renaissance has been particularly significant given our growing understanding of how fermented foods may support cognitive health and longevity through their impact on the gut-brain axis.

By following these science-based safety protocols while honoring traditional fermentation wisdom, we can create nutrient-rich foods that may contribute to both our longevity and cognitive vitality. The key lies in maintaining a careful balance between promoting beneficial bacterial growth while preventing the proliferation of harmful microorganisms - a practice that bridges ancient food preservation techniques with modern health objectives.As we conclude our exploration of fermentation's role in longevity and health, it's remarkable to reflect on how far we've come in understanding these ancient preservation techniques. Our ancestors, who often lived only into their 40s or 50s due to various health challenges including foodborne illnesses and nutritional deficiencies, unknowingly developed preservation methods that would eventually contribute to our increased longevity. Today, we understand that fermented foods not only preserve nutrients but enhance them, creating powerful allies for both gut and brain health.

The journey from necessity-driven food preservation to scientifically-validated health practice mirrors humanity's broader progression in understanding nutrition and longevity. What began as a simple means of survival has emerged as a sophisticated tool for promoting health and extending lifespan. The traditional wisdom of fermentation, passed down through generations, has been validated by modern science, revealing benefits that extend far beyond basic food preservation.

Through this chapter, we've explored how different cultures developed unique fermentation practices, each contributing to the remarkable longevity observed in their populations. From Korean kimchi to Caucasian kefir, these traditional methods have not only preserved food but enhanced its nutritional value in ways that support both physical and cognitive health. The microbiome connection, in particular, has emerged as a crucial link between fermented foods and longevity, offering new insights into how these ancient practices contribute to modern wellness.

We've also discovered how traditional preservation techniques can be adapted for contemporary use while maintaining their core benefits. The story of Blake, who transformed his health through traditional fermentation practices, illustrates how these ancient methods can address modern health challenges. His journey from chronic health issues to vibrant well-being exemplifies the potential these practices hold for our own longevity goals.

As we look to the future, the integration of traditional fermentation wisdom with modern scientific understanding offers exciting possibilities for extending both lifespan and healthspan. By incorporating these time-tested practices into our daily lives, we can harness the power of beneficial microorganisms to support our health and longevity in ways our ancestors could never have imagined.

Remember that the path to longevity isn't about discovering new miracle solutions, but often about rediscovering and properly implementing the wisdom our ancestors left us. Through careful attention to traditional fermentation practices and modern safety protocols, we can create nutrient-rich foods that support our journey toward optimal health and longevity. The key lies in maintaining a balance between honoring ancient wisdom and embracing scientific understanding - a synthesis that offers powerful tools for extending and enriching our lives.

As you begin your own fermentation journey, remember that every culture you nurture, every batch you prepare, connects you to an unbroken chain of human wisdom stretching back thousands of years. This connection not only enriches our understanding of food preservation but provides practical tools for enhancing our health and longevity in the modern world. The art of fermentation truly stands as a bridge between past and present, offering timeless solutions for contemporary health challenges.

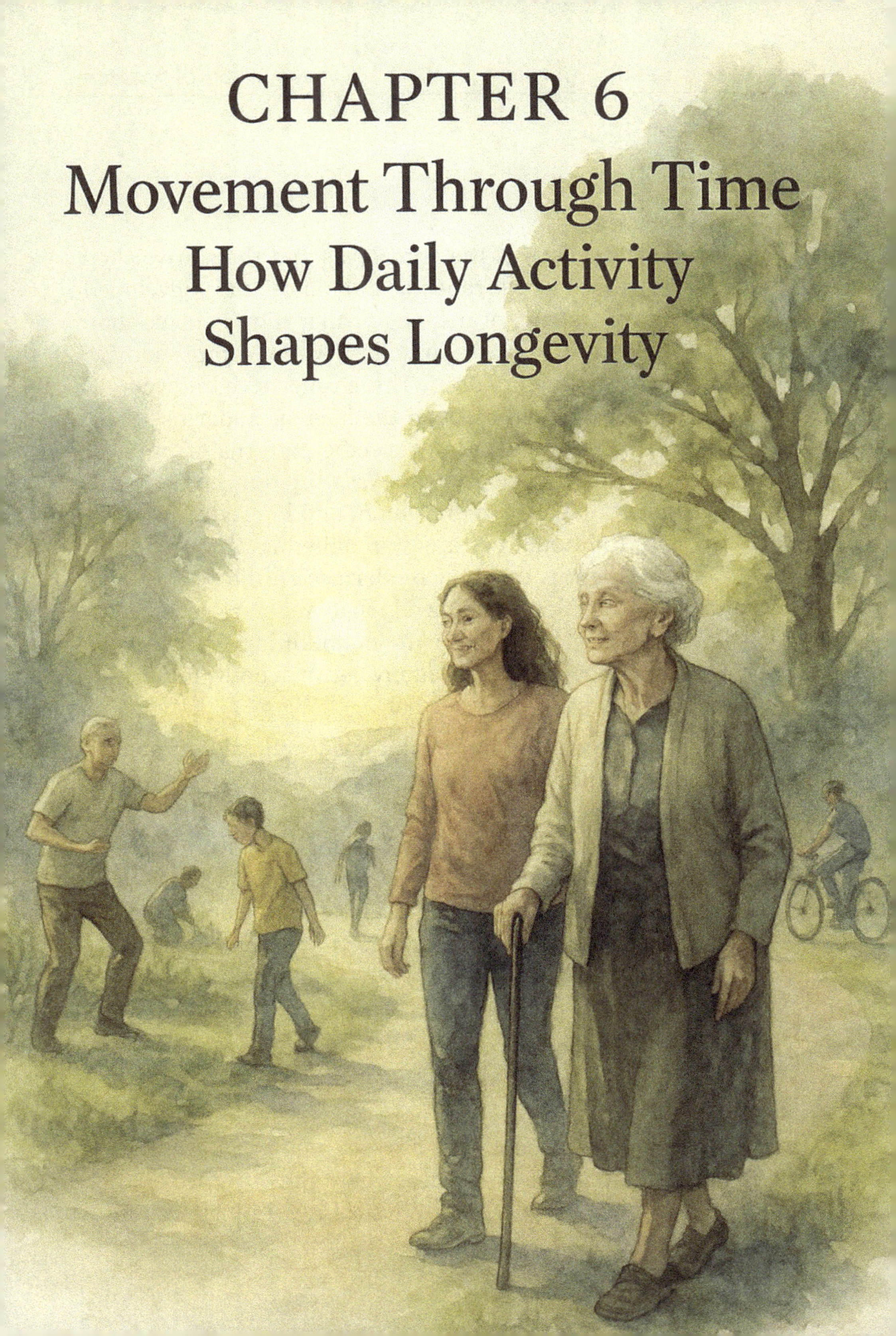

CHAPTER 6
Movement Through Time
How Daily Activity
Shapes Longevity

In the ancient valleys of the Himalayas and the sun-washed shores of the Mediterranean, our ancestors developed sophisticated systems of movement that did far more than simply keep them fit - these practices were comprehensive approaches to extending life itself. These time-tested movement traditions, when examined through the lens of modern science, reveal profound insights into how specific patterns of physical activity can activate longevity pathways in our bodies. The profound connection between movement and longevity has been understood by traditional cultures for millennia, though often through different lenses than our modern scientific perspective. These ancient societies recognized that regular, purposeful movement was not merely about maintaining strength or endurance, but about creating harmony between body, mind, and the natural world around them.

In many traditional cultures, movement was seamlessly woven into the fabric of daily life. Rather than compartmentalizing exercise into designated time slots, our ancestors engaged in constant, varied movement patterns throughout their days - from tending crops and carrying water to participating in communal dances and ritual ceremonies. This natural integration of movement into daily life offers valuable lessons for our modern approach to physical activity.

During my research into movement traditions, I became familiar with Maya, a former desk-bound professional who transformed her life by embracing ancient movement practices. At fifty, Maya was experiencing chronic back pain and declining mobility despite regular gym sessions. Her turning point came during a visit to a traditional village in Greece, where she observed elderly residents maintaining remarkable physical capabilities well into their 90s. Intrigued, she began studying their daily movement patterns - the way they squatted to tend gardens, carried water jugs on their heads, and participated in traditional dances. Maya spent the next year documenting and practicing these natural movement patterns, gradually incorporating them into her daily routine. She learned to replace her rigid gym schedule with more natural, flowing movements throughout the day. She began walking on uneven terrain, carrying groceries home instead of driving, and practicing traditional dance movements. Within six months, her back pain disappeared, her posture improved, and her overall mobility increased significantly. Now at 55, Maya teaches others how to incorporate these ancestral movement patterns into modern life, showing that the secret to lasting physical vitality might lie not in modern exercise machines, but in returning to the fundamental movements that kept our ancestors strong and mobile throughout their lives.

This transformative story illustrates a crucial principle: our bodies are designed for diverse, continuous movement rather than the sedentary lifestyle punctuated by intense exercise that has become common in modern society. Traditional movement practices offer us a window into how we can better align our physical activity with our body's natural capabilities and needs.

As we explore these ancient movement traditions, we'll discover how they not only enhanced physical capabilities but also promoted mental clarity, emotional balance, and social connection. From the flowing movements of tai chi to the grounding practices of traditional farming communities, these time-tested approaches to physical activity offer valuable insights for modern life.

In this chapter, we'll examine how various cultures developed sophisticated systems of movement that promoted longevity, and more importantly, how we can adapt these practices to enhance our own lives. We'll explore the science behind why these traditional movement patterns are so effective and provide practical ways to incorporate them into our daily routines, regardless of age or current fitness level.

Natural Movement Patterns: The Foundation of Longevity Exercise

Throughout human history, our bodies evolved for constant, varied movement - hunting, gathering, farming, and performing daily tasks that required strength, agility, and endurance[58][60]. This natural movement pattern was disrupted by the industrial revolution and modern conveniences, leading to increasingly sedentary lifestyles that our ancestors would hardly recognize. Yet within these ancient movement patterns lies a profound secret to longevity that modern science is now validating.

Research from the world's Blue Zones, particularly Okinawa and Sardinia, reveals that natural movement patterns remain central to the exceptional longevity of their inhabitants[58][59]. These communities don't rely on gym memberships or structured exercise programs. Instead, they maintain their vitality through constant, purposeful movement integrated seamlessly into daily life - gardening, walking on uneven terrain, carrying water, and performing household tasks that require squatting, lifting, and reaching.

The fundamental natural movement patterns that promote longevity include squatting, which maintains lower body strength and balance; lunging, which enhances stability and mobility; pushing and pulling movements that preserve upper body function; and the essential practice of walking[57][58][60]. These movements train the body across all three anatomical planes - sagittal (forward/backward), frontal (side-to-side), and transverse (rotational) - ensuring comprehensive functional fitness that supports independence as we age[60].

Modern research has demonstrated that these natural movement patterns do more than just maintain physical capability - they actually activate longevity pathways in our bodies. Regular engagement in these movements has been shown to improve immune function, enhance sleep quality, increase bone density, and support cardiovascular health[58] [59]. Perhaps most significantly, natural movement patterns have been linked to improved cognitive function and neuroplasticity, helping to prevent age-related cognitive decline[59].

The key to incorporating these longevity-promoting movements lies not in trying to replicate exactly how our ancestors moved, but in understanding the principles behind their movement patterns and adapting them to modern life. For instance, squatting to tend a garden can be replicated through bodyweight squats while waiting for coffee to brew. The natural pulling motions used in traditional farming can be mimicked through rowing exercises or resistance band work[58] [60].

In Okinawa, one of the world's most studied Blue Zones, elderly residents maintain a tradition of sitting and rising from the floor multiple times daily - a practice that combines several natural movement patterns and has been correlated with longer life expectancy[58]. This simple yet profound habit requires strength, balance, and mobility, serving as a practical test of functional fitness.

To incorporate these movement patterns into modern life, focus on mastering fundamental exercises that mirror ancestral movements. Start with basic squats and lunges, progressing to carrying exercises like farmer's walks, and include rotational movements that maintain spine health and coordination[57] [60]. The goal isn't to achieve perfect form immediately, but to gradually build competency in these essential movement patterns.

Importantly, natural movement patterns should be practiced consistently rather than intensely. Research shows that frequent, moderate engagement in these movements yields greater longevity benefits than sporadic intense exercise[57] [59]. This aligns with traditional practices in long-lived communities, where movement is a constant, gentle presence in daily life rather than a scheduled burst of active.

The cognitive benefits of natural movement patterns cannot be overstated. Walking, particularly in nature, has been shown to boost brain-derived neurotrophic factor (BDNF), a protein crucial for neural health and cognitive function[59]. The complex coordination required in natural movement patterns also challenges the brain, creating new neural pathways and supporting cognitive resilience as we age.

By returning to these fundamental movement patterns, we're not just exercising - we're reconnecting with our evolutionary heritage and activating ancient pathways to longevity[58][60]. The key is to view movement not as something we do for 30 minutes at the gym, but as an essential, integrated aspect of daily life, just as our longest-lived ancestors have done for generations.

Traditional Strength Practices: From Farmer's Walks to Functional Training

Long before the advent of modern gyms and fitness equipment, our ancestors developed remarkable strength through their daily activities. Traditional strength practices, deeply rooted in agricultural and survival tasks, have proven to be some of the most

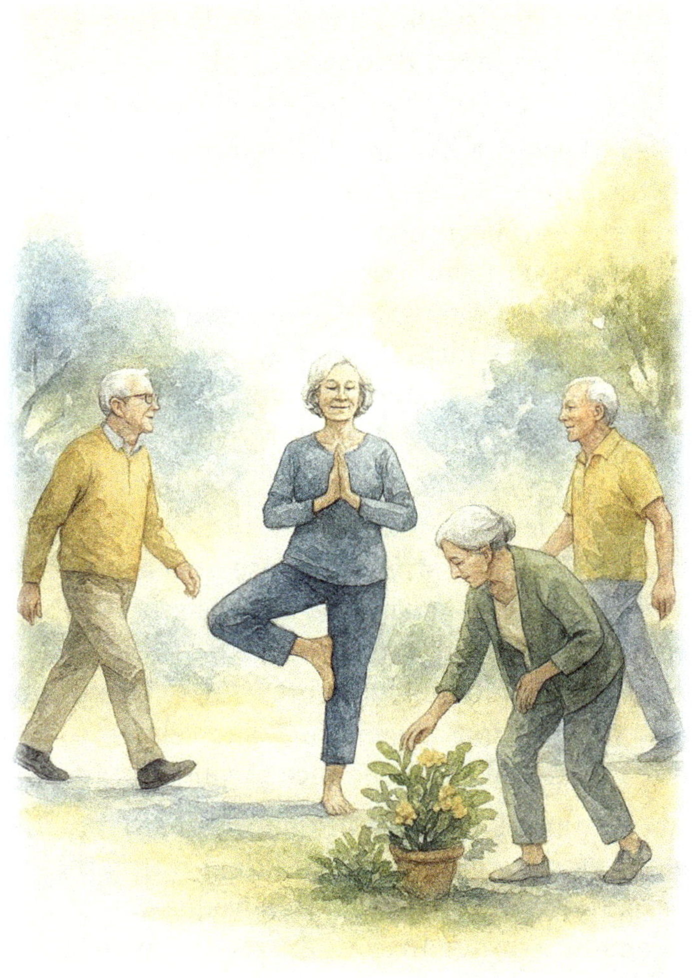

effective methods for building functional strength and promoting longevity. These time-tested movements, particularly the farmer's walk and other load-carrying exercises, activate multiple muscle groups simultaneously while improving cardiovascular health and bone density[61][62].

The farmer's walk, a fundamental movement pattern that involves carrying heavy weights while walking, emerged from the practical demands of agricultural life. Research has shown that this seemingly simple exercise engages nearly every major muscle group in the body, from the legs and core to the upper back and forearms[61][62]. Modern studies have revealed that grip strength, which is heavily developed through carrying exercises, serves as a powerful predictor of overall health and longevity[62][63].

What makes these traditional strength practices particularly valuable is their direct correlation to functional independence as we age. Dr. Peter Attia, a prominent longevity expert, emphasizes that the ability to perform loaded carries is "a strong indicator that you'll retain the strength needed in your last decades to handle everyday tasks like carrying groceries or opening jars—crucial for staying independent."[64] This practical application of strength has profound implications for maintaining quality of life as we age.

The physiological benefits of these traditional movements extend far beyond mere muscle strength. Research has demonstrated that exercises like the farmer's walk significantly improve cardiovascular fitness, enhance bone density, and promote proper posture and spinal alignment[61][62][64][65]. These benefits are particularly crucial for preventing age-related decline and maintaining functional independence throughout life[63].

Perhaps most remarkably, traditional strength practices have been shown to support cognitive health through their complex movement patterns and coordination requirements. The full-body engagement required in these exercises increases blood flow to the brain and stimulates the production of neural growth factors, potentially helping to prevent age-related cognitive decline[61][62].

In the context of modern life, these ancestral strength practices offer a refreshing alternative to complicated exercise routines. Their simplicity and accessibility make them ideal for people of all ages and fitness levels[64]. Physical therapists have observed that older adults who regularly incorporate loaded carries into their routines maintain better mobility and confidence in their daily activities[63].

The metabolic impact of traditional strength practices is equally impressive. By engaging multiple large muscle groups simultaneously, these movements create a significant metabolic response that continues long after the exercise is complete. This effect, known as excess post-exercise oxygen consumption (EPOC), contributes to improved body composition and metabolic health[62].

To incorporate these traditional strength practices into modern life, focus on progressive loading and consistent practice rather than maximum weight. Begin with manageable loads and gradually increase the weight and distance as strength improves. The goal is to build functional strength that translates to real-world activities, not to achieve arbitrary numbers on a scale[62][64].

Importantly, these traditional strength practices support joint health through their emphasis on natural movement patterns. Unlike isolated machine exercises, functional movements like the farmer's walk train the body to work as an integrated unit, promoting better coordination and reducing the risk of injury[62][65]. This comprehensive approach to strength training aligns perfectly with our evolutionary heritage and the way our bodies were designed to move.

The wisdom of traditional strength practices lies in their simplicity and effectiveness. By returning to these fundamental movement patterns, we can tap into a proven method of building strength, enhancing longevity, and maintaining independence throughout our lives. As modern research continues to validate the benefits of these ancestral practices, their relevance to contemporary health and fitness becomes increasingly clear[62] [63] [64].

Mobility and Joint Health: Ancient Techniques for Modern Bodies

Ancient civilizations understood something profound about joint health and mobility that modern science is now validating - the human body requires consistent, mindful movement to maintain its vitality well into advanced age. From the flowing postures of Indian yoga to the deliberate movements of Chinese Tai Chi, traditional cultures developed sophisticated practices for preserving joint function and mobility that remain remarkably relevant today.

In Okinawa, one of the world's most studied Blue Zones, centenarians maintain extraordinary mobility well past 100 years through daily practices that emphasize natural movement patterns[27] [11]. They regularly sit on the floor and rise without using their hands, garden in positions that require deep squatting, and participate in traditional dances that incorporate gentle rotational movements. These activities, performed consistently over decades, help maintain synovial fluid production, balance muscle pairs, and enhance proprioception - all critical factors in joint longevity.

Modern research has revealed that these ancient movement traditions work through multiple physiological pathways to support joint health. When we perform slow, mindful movements like those found in Tai Chi and yoga, we stimulate the production of synovial fluid that nourishes cartilage and reduces friction in our joints. These practices also help balance the muscles around our joints, ensuring proper alignment and reducing unnecessary wear and tear.

The anti-inflammatory effects of traditional movement practices are particularly noteworthy. Studies of long-lived populations show that regular, moderate movement helps reduce systemic inflammation - a key driver of joint degeneration and many age-related conditions[11]. This understanding aligns perfectly with ancient wisdom that emphasized daily, gentle movement over sporadic intense exercise.

In the mountainous regions of Sardinia, elderly shepherds demonstrate the remarkable preservation of joint health through natural movement patterns[27]. Their daily routines involve walking on varied terrain, which engages joints through multiple planes of motion while building strength and balance. This real-world example shows how traditional lifestyle patterns can maintain mobility well into advanced age.

For modern individuals seeking to incorporate these time-tested practices, the key lies in consistency rather than intensity[11]. Begin by introducing gentle movement patterns throughout your day - practice rising from a chair without using your hands, take short walks on natural terrain, or explore basic yoga poses that emphasize joint mobility. The goal is to create a sustainable practice that can be maintained for decades, just as our longest-lived ancestors have done.

Traditional Ayurvedic and Chinese medicine also offer valuable insights into joint health through their emphasis on manual therapies and massage. These practices, when combined with mindful movement, help maintain joint flexibility while promoting circulation and reducing stiffness. Modern research confirms that regular manual therapy can significantly improve range of motion and joint function.

Perhaps most importantly, these ancient practices recognize the profound connection between mind and body in maintaining joint health. The mindful awareness cultivated through traditional movement practices enhances proprioception - our body's ability to sense position and movement - which is crucial for preventing injuries and maintaining mobility as we age.

By adapting these ancient wisdom traditions to modern life, we can create a comprehensive approach to joint health that supports longevity. The key is to view movement not as something we do occasionally, but as an essential daily practice that maintains our body's natural capabilities. Just as our ancestors understood, regular, mindful movement is the foundation of lasting mobility and joint health.

Rhythmic Movement and Cardiovascular Health: Dancing Through the Ages

Throughout human history, dance has been more than just a form of artistic expression - it has served as a powerful tool for maintaining cardiovascular health and promoting longevity. In regions with high concentrations of centenarians, particularly the Blue Zones of Sardinia, Okinawa, and Ikaria, communal dancing remains deeply woven into the fabric of daily life[27][11], offering profound insights into the connection between rhythmic movement and extended lifespan.

The relationship between dance and cardiovascular health has been extensively studied, with remarkable findings. Research published in the American Journal of Preventive Medicine revealed that adults who regularly engaged in dance activities had a 46% lower risk of cardiovascular mortality compared to non-dancers, even after accounting for other forms of physical activity. This striking statistic suggests that the unique combination of physical movement, social engagement, and cognitive stimulation inherent in dance may offer protective benefits beyond traditional exercise.

In Sardinia, the traditional folk dance "ballu tundu" exemplifies how rhythmic movement has been preserved through generations as both a cultural practice and a health-promoting activity. This circular dance, performed by all age groups during festivals and celebrations, combines aerobic exercise with social connection - two critical factors consistently observed among centenarians[27]. The dance's continuous, moderate-intensity movements help maintain cardiovascular fitness while fostering the community bonds that research has linked to increased longevity.

The physiological benefits of dance extend beyond heart health. Regular participation in rhythmic movement has been shown to improve circulation, enhance oxygen delivery throughout the body, and reduce blood pressure and cholesterol levels. Perhaps most significantly, dance engages multiple body systems simultaneously, creating a comprehensive workout that builds strength, balance, and coordination while maintaining joint mobility.

The cognitive benefits of dance are equally impressive. The complex patterns and movements involved in dancing challenge the brain's neuroplasticity, potentially helping to prevent cognitive decline. This mental engagement, combined with the social aspects of group dancing, creates a powerful cocktail for brain health that aligns with findings from the New England Centenarian Study[66] regarding the importance of maintaining both physical and mental activity throughout life.

In Blue Zone communities, where dancing remains a near-universal pastime, researchers have observed that this practice helps maintain vitality well into advanced age. Dan Buettner's extensive research into these longevity hotspots consistently highlights how regular, rhythmic movement through dance serves as both a social connector and a natural form of exercise that people continue to enjoy throughout their lives.

The accessibility of dance as a form of exercise makes it particularly valuable for promoting population-wide health. Unlike many forms of exercise that require special equipment or facilities, dance can be adapted for all ages and ability levels, making it an inclusive activity that can be maintained throughout life. This accessibility aligns with recommendations from major health organizations, including the World Health Organization and American Heart Association, which emphasize the importance of regular, moderate-intensity aerobic activity.

The social dimension of dance cannot be overstated in its contribution to longevity. Group dances create opportunities for regular social interaction, which studies have consistently shown to be a crucial factor in maintaining both physical and mental health as we age[11]. This social engagement helps combat isolation and depression while providing the motivation to remain physically active.

For those seeking to incorporate dance into their longevity practices, the key lies in consistency rather than intensity. Regular, moderate engagement in rhythmic movement, whether through formal dance classes or informal social dancing, can provide the cardiovascular benefits while minimizing the risk of injury or burnout. This approach mirrors the traditional practices observed in long-lived communities, where dance is viewed not as a workout but as an integral part of daily life.

The evidence supporting dance as a longevity-promoting activity continues to grow. From its ability to maintain cardiovascular health and cognitive function to its role in fostering social connections, dance embodies many of the key factors that research has identified as crucial for healthy aging. As we seek to understand and implement the secrets of centenarians[11], the incorporation of regular rhythmic movement through dance stands out as one of the most accessible and enjoyable paths to extended healthspan.

Balance and Coordination: Time-Tested Practices for Aging Well

Among the most remarkable attributes of centenarians in Blue Zone regions is their exceptional balance and coordination well into advanced age. In Okinawa, elders maintain an active lifestyle that naturally incorporates balance-challenging activities, from tending their gardens to participating in traditional dance movements[27]. This preservation of balance and coordination isn't merely about preventing falls - though that's certainly important - it represents a fundamental aspect of healthy aging that modern science is now validating with compelling research.

The New England Centenarian Study has revealed that individuals who maintain good balance and coordination throughout their lives tend to experience better overall health outcomes and increased independence in their later years[66]. This finding aligns perfectly with observations from traditional cultures where daily activities naturally challenge and maintain these crucial physical capabilities.

In Sardinia's mountain villages, where some of the world's oldest populations reside, elders continue to navigate steep, uneven terrain well into their nineties[27][11]. Their remarkable balance and coordination stem not from formal exercise programs but from lifelong habits of walking on challenging surfaces and performing manual tasks that require complex movement patterns. These natural movement practices have been shown to activate multiple neural pathways, contributing to both physical stability and cognitive resilience.

Modern research has demonstrated that balance and coordination training does more than just prevent falls - it actually stimulates neuroplasticity, the brain's ability to form new neural connections. This process is crucial for maintaining cognitive function and may help explain why populations that maintain these physical capabilities often exhibit lower rates of age-related cognitive decline.

The practice of Tai Chi, particularly prevalent among long-lived populations in Asia, offers a perfect example of how traditional movement patterns can enhance balance and coordination. Studies have shown that regular Tai Chi practice significantly improves postural control and reduces fall risk in older adults. The slow, deliberate movements characteristic of this ancient practice challenge the body's proprioceptive system while promoting mind-body connection.

In traditional societies, balance and coordination were naturally maintained through daily activities like carrying water, tending livestock, and participating in communal dances[11]. Today, we must be more intentional about incorporating these movement patterns into our lives. Simple practices like standing on one leg while brushing teeth or walking on uneven surfaces can help maintain these crucial physical abilities.

The connection between balance, coordination, and longevity extends beyond physical safety. These capabilities allow older adults to remain physically active, which correlates strongly with longer, healthier lives[11]. In Blue Zone communities, the ability to participate in physical activities well into advanced age helps preserve social connections and sense of purpose, or what Okinawans call "ikigai"[27].

Practical implementation of balance and coordination training doesn't require expensive equipment or complicated routines. Walking on varied terrain, practicing simple balance exercises, and engaging in traditional movement practices like dance or Tai Chi can all contribute to maintaining these vital capabilities. The key is consistency rather than intensity - regular, moderate challenges to balance and coordination appear to yield the greatest benefits for longevity.

Importantly, these practices should begin well before advanced age. Research indicates that maintaining balance and coordination throughout life creates a physical reserve that becomes crucial in later years. This aligns with observations from centenarian populations, where lifelong movement patterns contribute to remarkable physical capabilities in advanced age.

The wisdom of traditional cultures in maintaining balance and coordination offers valuable lessons for modern aging. By incorporating these time-tested practices into our daily routines, we can build and maintain the physical capabilities that support independence and vitality throughout life. Whether through traditional movement practices, mindful walking, or simple balance challenges, these fundamental aspects of physical function remain crucial to healthy aging and longevity.Throughout this chapter, we've explored how movement traditions from across the globe have contributed to human longevity and vitality. From the natural movement patterns of agricultural communities to the sophisticated practices of ancient movement traditions, we've discovered that the key to physical longevity often lies in returning to the fundamental ways our bodies were designed to move.

The stark contrast between historical and modern lifespans becomes particularly evident when we examine movement patterns. Our ancestors, despite their constant physical activity, often lived shorter lives due to infectious diseases, harsh living conditions, and limited medical knowledge. However, their movement practices - when combined with modern medical advances and improved living conditions - offer powerful insights into extending not just our lifespan, but our healthspan.

The research we've explored shows that traditional movement practices do more than just maintain physical health - they play a crucial role in preserving cognitive function and preventing neurodegenerative conditions. The complex coordination required in traditional dance forms, the mindful awareness developed through practices like Tai Chi, and the neural engagement demanded by natural movement patterns all contribute to brain health and cognitive resilience.

Perhaps most significantly, we've learned that longevity through movement isn't about intense, sporadic exercise but rather about consistent, varied, and purposeful physical activity integrated naturally into daily life. The centenarians in Blue Zones demonstrate this principle perfectly - they maintain their vitality not through rigid exercise programs but through constant, gentle movement woven seamlessly into their daily routines.

As we've seen through Maya's story and countless others, the adaptation of ancient movement practices to modern life doesn't require a complete lifestyle overhaul. Small, consistent changes - like incorporating natural movement patterns, traditional strength practices, or regular dance sessions - can significantly impact our long-term health and longevity.

The key takeaway from this exploration of movement traditions is clear: our bodies thrive on regular, varied movement that engages both physical and cognitive functions. By understanding and implementing these time-tested practices in ways that fit our modern lives, we can tap into the same longevity-promoting benefits that have sustained healthy populations for generations.

As we move forward, let's remember that the goal isn't to perfectly replicate ancient movement patterns but to understand their principles and adapt them meaningfully to our contemporary lives. Whether through carrying groceries home instead of driving, practicing traditional dance forms, or incorporating natural movement patterns into our daily routines, we can all find ways to harness the longevity-promoting power of movement.

In the next chapter, we'll explore how the mind-body connection, understood through various cultural traditions, plays a crucial role in stress management and overall longevity. We'll discover how ancient wisdom about the interconnectedness of mental and physical health aligns with modern scientific understanding, providing us with powerful tools for enhancing our well-being and extending our healthspan.

The Mind-Body Connection

How Inner Peace Supports Longevity

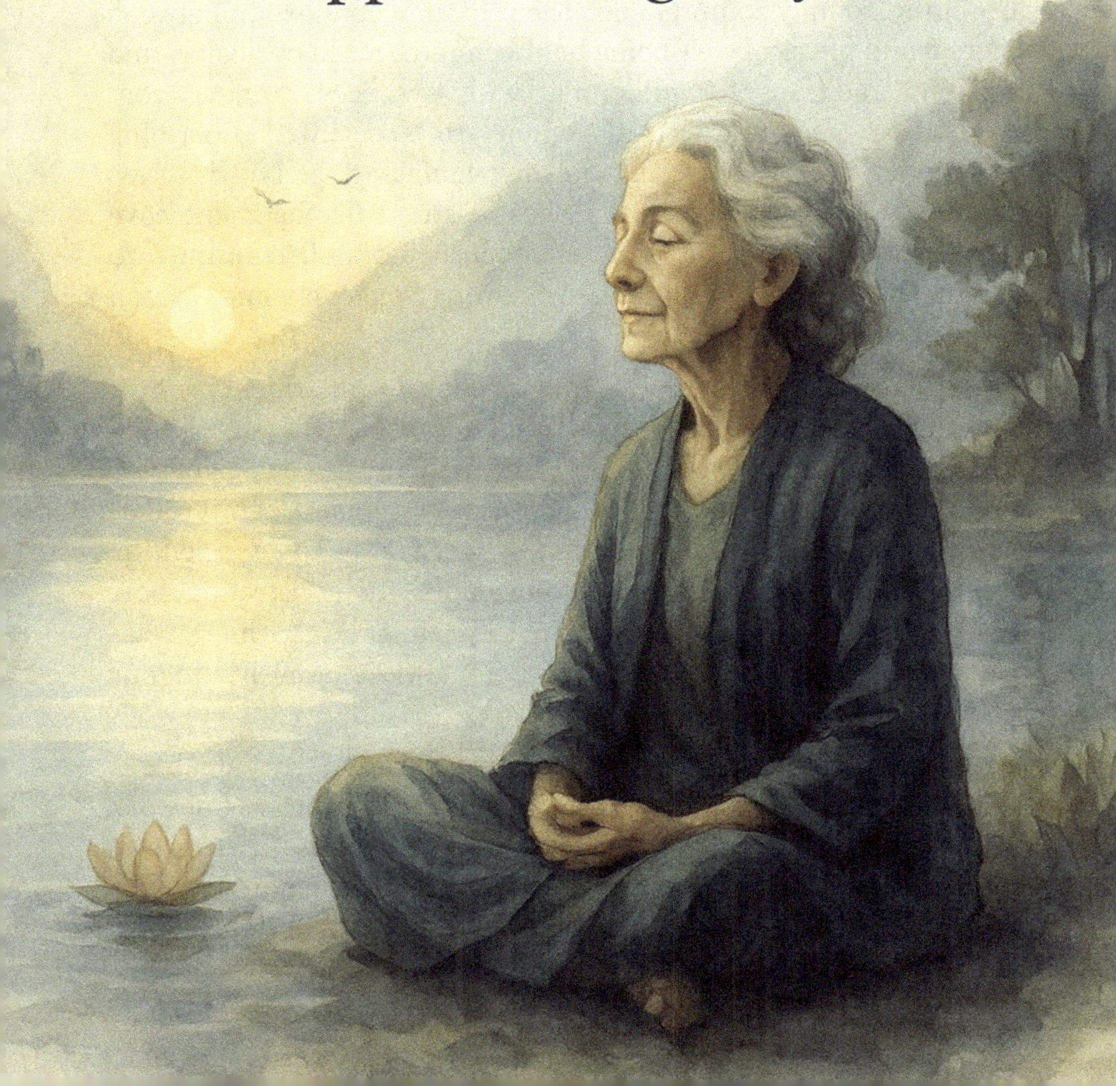

Nestled in the ancient practices of cultures spanning from the meditation halls of Tibet to the healing centers of ancient Greece lies a profound understanding of how our mental state influences our physical health. These time-tested traditions, developed over centuries of careful observation and practice, reveal sophisticated approaches to managing the delicate balance between mind and body that modern science is only now beginning to fully comprehend. The profound connection between mental and physical well-being has been recognized by healers and wisdom traditions for millennia, with practices ranging from meditation and mindful movement to specialized breathing techniques offering powerful tools for managing the body's stress response. These ancient approaches to stress management have proven remarkably prescient, as modern research continues to validate their effectiveness in promoting longevity and overall health.

Across diverse cultures, we find striking similarities in how traditional societies understood and addressed the mind-body relationship. From the traditional Chinese medicine concept of qi to the Indian understanding of prana, these systems recognized that mental state profoundly influences physical health. Today, scientific research has confirmed these connections, demonstrating how chronic stress can accelerate aging at the cellular level, while stress-management practices can activate longevity pathways in our bodies.

What makes these traditional approaches particularly valuable is their holistic nature - they don't simply address symptoms but work to restore balance to the entire system. The Japanese practice of shinrin-yoku (forest bathing), for instance, doesn't just reduce stress hormones; it enhances immune function and promotes cardiovascular health. Similarly, traditional breathing practices don't merely calm the mind; they influence heart rate variability, inflammation levels, and cellular repair mechanisms.

During my research into traditional stress management practices, I met Sophia, a former emergency room nurse who had reached a breaking point from chronic workplace stress. Despite her medical background, conventional stress management techniques weren't providing the relief she needed. Her journey led her to explore traditional practices from various cultures, beginning with Japanese forest bathing (shinrin-yoku). She started spending her days off immersed in nature, practicing the slow, mindful walking and breathing techniques that had been used for centuries in Japan. Gradually, she incorporated other traditional practices - Thai chi in the mornings, Tibetan singing bowl meditation in the evenings, and Indian pranayama breathing techniques during her work breaks. The transformation was remarkable. Her cortisol levels normalized, her sleep improved, and she developed a new resilience to workplace stress. Most surprisingly, she found that these ancient practices not only helped her personally but also enhanced her ability to care for patients, as she began teaching simple breathing techniques to those in acute distress. Sophia's experience demonstrated how ancient wisdom could provide practical solutions to modern stress, bridging the gap between traditional practices and contemporary healthcare needs.

What's particularly fascinating about these traditional stress management techniques is their accessibility and adaptability. While modern life presents unique challenges our ancestors never faced - from digital overwhelm to 24/7 work cultures - the fundamental principles of these ancient practices remain surprisingly relevant. They offer practical tools for managing stress that can be adapted to fit contemporary lifestyles while maintaining their core benefits.

As we delve deeper into this chapter, we'll explore specific techniques from various cultures, examining how they work from both traditional and scientific perspectives. We'll learn how to adapt these practices for modern life without losing their essential benefits, and discover how different approaches can be combined to create a comprehensive stress management strategy. Most importantly, we'll see how these ancient wisdom traditions can help us navigate the unique challenges of our modern world while promoting longevity and vibrant health.

Traditional Breathing Techniques and Their Impact on the Nervous System

Among the most profound discoveries in longevity research is how something as simple as conscious breathing can dramatically impact our nervous system and overall health. Ancient wisdom traditions have long understood this connection, developing sophisticated breathing techniques that modern science now validates as powerful tools for extending both lifespan and healthspan.

The practice of controlled breathing, known as pranayama in the yogic tradition, has been shown to activate what scientists call the parasympathetic nervous system - our body's natural "rest and digest" mode[67] [68]. This activation triggers a cascade of beneficial physiological responses that our ancestors inherently understood, even without the scientific terminology we use today. When we engage in slow, deliberate breathing practices like diaphragmatic breathing or the 4-7-8 technique, we essentially hack into our nervous system's control panel, manually switching from stress mode to relaxation mode[67].

Research has shown that specific breathing patterns can significantly impact our brain's function and structure. For instance, the practice of coherent breathing - maintaining a steady rate of about 5-6 breaths per minute - has been demonstrated to increase Heart Rate Variability (HRV), a key marker of longevity and stress resilience[69]. This practice helps balance the autonomic nervous system, reducing inflammation and supporting cellular repair mechanisms throughout the body[68].

One particularly fascinating technique that has gained scientific attention is alternate nostril breathing, or Nadi Shodhana. This ancient practice, which involves breathing through one nostril at a time, has been shown to balance the activity between the brain's hemispheres and reduce stress levels measurably[67] [68]. Studies have documented how this technique can lower blood pressure, reduce cortisol levels, and improve cognitive function - all factors that contribute to increased longevity[68] [69].

The power of cyclic sighing, a technique involving a double inhale followed by a prolonged exhalation, has recently emerged as one of the most effective breathing practices for mood enhancement and stress reduction. Research has shown that this particular pattern of breathing can lead to greater improvements in mood and reduction in negative emotions than traditional mindfulness meditation alone[70]. This finding provides a tangible link between ancient breathing practices and modern emotional wellness.

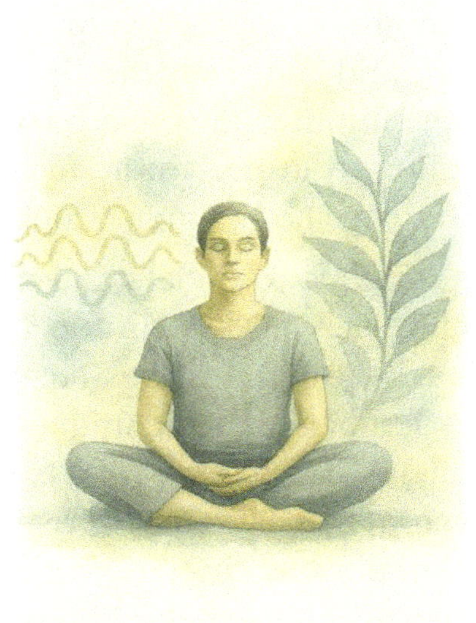

For those seeking to incorporate these techniques into daily life, the box breathing method offers a structured approach that's both powerful and accessible. This technique, which involves equal-length phases of inhalation, hold, exhalation, and hold, has been adopted by military special forces for its remarkable ability to maintain composure under extreme stress. The practice follows a simple 4-4-4-4 pattern: inhale for four counts, hold for four, exhale for four, and hold for four before beginning again[67].

What makes these breathing techniques particularly valuable for longevity is their cumulative effect on the body's stress response systems. Chronic stress accelerates aging at the cellular level, but regular practice of these ancient breathing methods has been shown to counteract this effect[68][69]. Through improved oxygenation and nervous system regulation, these practices support the body's natural repair mechanisms and help maintain the length of telomeres - the protective caps on our chromosomes that are associated with longevity[68].

The beauty of these traditional breathing practices lies in their simplicity and accessibility. Unlike many modern interventions, they require no special equipment or facilities, yet their benefits are profound and scientifically verified[67][68][69]. Whether practiced for a few minutes during a busy workday or as part of a longer meditation routine, these techniques offer a direct path to activating our body's innate longevity mechanisms.

As we continue to understand the intricate connections between breathing, nervous system function, and longevity, these ancient practices reveal themselves not just as stress management tools, but as fundamental techniques for extending healthspan and lifespan[69][70]. By incorporating these time-tested methods into our daily routines, we tap into a wisdom that bridges the gap between ancient understanding and modern science, offering a practical approach to enhancing both the quality and quantity of our years.

Movement Meditation: From Tai Chi to Walking Practices

Among the most profound discoveries in longevity research is how mindful movement practices can serve as powerful tools for extending both lifespan and healthspan. Ancient wisdom traditions recognized that combining physical activity with mental focus created uniquely beneficial effects on health and longevity - an insight that modern science now validates through extensive research.

Tai Chi, often described as "meditation in motion," stands as one of the most well-studied movement meditation practices[71][72]. This ancient Chinese art seamlessly blends physical exercise with mindfulness, making it accessible across ages and fitness levels[74]. Research has shown that regular Tai Chi practice can significantly reduce stress and anxiety, with some studies suggesting it may be even more effective than conventional exercise due to its meditative components[71][72]. "Tai chi incorporates deep breathing and mindful focus, which helps calm the nervous system and reduce stress," explains Dr. Jenelle Kim, a doctor of Chinese Medicine[72].

The health benefits of Tai Chi extend far beyond stress reduction. Studies have demonstrated its remarkable impact on cognitive function, particularly in older adults, where it has been shown to enhance memory and executive function, and even increase brain size in some cases[71][74]. This cognitive enhancement may be particularly significant given our modern understanding of brain plasticity and its role in healthy aging. Additionally, Tai Chi consistently improves balance and coordination, reducing fall risk - a crucial factor in maintaining independence and health as we age[71][72].

Walking meditation, another powerful form of movement meditation, offers similar benefits while being perhaps even more accessible than Tai Chi. Found in many traditions, including Buddhism and modern mindfulness programs, walking meditation involves bringing full attention to the simple act of walking. This practice grounds attention in the present moment, interrupting cycles of rumination and worry that can accelerate cellular aging through chronic stress activation.

The beauty of these movement meditation practices lies in their ability to simultaneously address multiple aspects of health.

While moving the body, they activate what scientists call the parasympathetic nervous system - our body's natural "rest and digest" mode. This activation triggers a cascade of beneficial physiological responses that support longevity, from reduced inflammation to enhanced cellular repair mechanisms.

What makes these practices particularly valuable for modern life is their adaptability. Unlike many traditional exercises that require specific equipment or environments, movement meditation can be practiced almost anywhere. A busy professional might incorporate mindful walking during their commute, while someone with limited mobility might practice modified Tai Chi movements from a seated position[71][72][74].

The integration of breath awareness with movement adds another dimension to these practices' longevity benefits. Deep, diaphragmatic breathing enhances oxygenation, lowers blood pressure, and supports relaxation[72][74]. When combined with mindful movement, this breathing practice becomes even more powerful, creating a synergistic effect that supports both physical and mental well-being.

Clinical programs incorporating these movement meditation practices have reported impressive results. Participants often experience improvements in blood pressure, sleep quality, and overall resilience[74]. For those dealing with chronic conditions such as fibromyalgia, COPD, Parkinson's disease, and heart disease, these practices have shown particular promise in improving quality of life and symptom management[71].

Perhaps most significantly, movement meditation practices appear to address one of the fundamental challenges of modern life - the disconnect between mind and body that often results from our increasingly sedentary and digitally-focused lifestyles. By bringing conscious awareness to physical movement, these practices help restore this vital connection, supporting not just longevity but also the quality of life throughout our extended years.

As we continue to understand the mechanisms behind these practices, their value becomes increasingly clear. They offer a practical approach to activating our body's innate longevity mechanisms[73] while providing immediate benefits for both physical and mental health. In a world where stress and disconnection often seem inevitable, these ancient practices offer a path to both immediate well-being and long-term health.

Sound Healing Traditions and Modern Stress Reduction

Throughout human history, cultures across the globe have recognized the profound impact of sound on human health and longevity[75,76,77,78]. From the resonant tones of Tibetan singing bowls echoing through Himalayan monasteries to the rhythmic vibrations of Aboriginal didgeridoos, these ancient practices have offered pathways to reduced stress, enhanced mental clarity, and improved overall well-being[77]. Modern science is now validating what our ancestors intuitively understood - that specific sound frequencies and patterns can fundamentally alter our physiological and psychological state.

The mechanisms behind sound healing's effectiveness are remarkably sophisticated. Research has shown that different organs and cells in our body maintain their own vibratory frequencies, and sound healing practices aim to restore equilibrium when these natural resonances become disrupted[76]. This understanding helps explain why traditional sound healing practices have persisted across millennia, offering benefits that extend beyond mere relaxation into the realm of cellular health and longevity.

Particularly noteworthy is the impact of sound healing on brainwave patterns. Through a process known as brainwave entrainment, rhythmic sounds can synchronize neural oscillations, effectively shifting the brain into states associated with deep relaxation, meditation, or restorative sleep[76][77]. This has profound implications for stress reduction and cognitive health, as chronic stress has been identified as a significant factor in accelerated aging and decreased longevity[75].

Clinical research has demonstrated that sound healing practices can trigger measurable physiological changes. Studies of Tibetan singing bowl meditation have shown significant decreases in tension, anxiety, and depression, with particularly notable benefits observed in adults aged 40-59[77]. These sessions have been associated with reductions in stress hormones like cortisol, while simultaneously promoting the activation of the parasympathetic nervous system - our body's natural "rest and digest" mode[77][79].

The accessibility of sound healing practices makes them particularly valuable in our modern context. Unlike many traditional health practices that require specific conditions or extensive training, sound healing can be adapted to various settings and needs[78]. From formal sound baths using multiple instruments to simple breathing practices accompanied by specific tones, these techniques offer flexible approaches to stress reduction and longevity enhancement[75][78].

Modern technology has expanded the reach of these ancient practices through digital adaptations like binaural beats - carefully crafted audio frequencies that present slightly different tones to each ear, creating a perceived third tone in the brain[76][77]. These contemporary innovations maintain the core principles of traditional sound healing while making them more accessible to today's busy lifestyles.

Perhaps most significantly, sound healing practices appear to address one of the fundamental challenges in promoting longevity - the need to reduce chronic stress while supporting cellular rejuvenation. Regular engagement with therapeutic sound practices may promote cellular health and mitigate the negative impacts of chronic stress, potentially contributing to increased lifespan[75]. This aligns with our growing understanding of how environmental factors, including sound, can influence our genetic expression and overall health trajectory.

The integration of sound healing into modern wellness practices represents a powerful synthesis of ancient wisdom and contemporary science[75][76][77][78]. As we continue to understand the mechanisms behind these practices, their value in promoting longevity becomes increasingly clear. Whether through traditional instruments, voice, or digital sound technology, these practices offer practical tools for managing stress, enhancing mental clarity, and supporting the body's natural healing processes - all crucial factors in extending both lifespan and healthspan[75][76][77][78][79].

Mind-Body Nutrition: Traditional Understanding of Food's Impact on Mental State

Ancient wisdom traditions across cultures have long recognized that food profoundly influences not just our physical health, but our mental and emotional well-being[27][11][66]. From the healing halls of Ayurvedic medicine to the traditional kitchens of Okinawa, our ancestors understood that the mind-body connection through nutrition was central to achieving both longevity and mental vitality[11].

In traditional Ayurvedic medicine, foods are carefully classified by their effects on the three doshas (Vata, Pitta, and Kapha), which influence both physical and mental states. Sattvic foods - fresh fruits, vegetables, whole grains, and nuts - are considered particularly beneficial for promoting mental clarity, emotional balance, and spiritual growth. This ancient understanding aligns remarkably well with modern research on the gut-brain axis, where we now know that certain nutrients and compounds directly influence neurotransmitter production and mental health.

The Traditional Chinese Medicine (TCM) approach offers another sophisticated framework for understanding food's impact on mental state. By categorizing foods according to their warming, cooling, or harmonizing properties, TCM practitioners have long prescribed specific dietary modifications to support emotional equilibrium and cognitive function. This system recognizes that different organs are connected to different emotions, and that supporting organ health through diet directly influences mental well-being.

Perhaps some of the most compelling evidence for the mind-body effects of nutrition comes from the world's Blue Zones, regions with the highest concentration of centenarians[27][11]. In Okinawa, Japan, the traditional diet rich in sweet potatoes, vegetables, tofu, and seaweed is accompanied by the practice of hara hachi bu - eating until only 80% full[27]. This mindful eating approach not only supports physical health but has been linked to improved mental clarity and reduced inflammation, both crucial factors in cognitive longevity.

The Mediterranean diet, another longevity-promoting eating pattern, demonstrates how certain nutritional combinations can specifically support brain health and emotional resilience. High in vegetables, fruits, whole grains, legumes, nuts, and olive oil, this diet has been associated with lower rates of depression and cognitive decline[11]. The abundance of antioxidants, omega-3 fatty acids, and polyphenols in these traditional foods provides direct support for brain health while reducing inflammation throughout the body.

Modern science has now validated these traditional understandings through research on the gut-brain axis, a sophisticated bidirectional communication system between our digestive tract and brain. We now know that the nutrients we consume influence the production of neurotransmitters like serotonin and dopamine, directly affecting our mood and cognitive function. The microbiota in our gut, influenced by our food choices, plays a crucial role in this communication system.

Particularly significant is the role of inflammation in mental health, a connection that traditional healing systems inherently understood. Diets high in processed foods and sugars can trigger chronic inflammation, which has been linked to both cognitive decline and mood disorders[11]. In contrast, the anti-inflammatory properties of traditional whole-food diets help support both mental clarity and emotional balance.

In centenarian communities, the mental benefits of traditional diets are often enhanced by social and cultural practices surrounding food. In Sardinia, Italy, meals are typically shared experiences that reduce stress and foster emotional well-being[11]. Similarly, in Ikaria, Greece, the daily ritual of preparing and sharing herbal teas made from sage, rosemary, and wild greens provides both nutritional and social benefits that support mental health.

The wisdom of these traditional approaches to mind-body nutrition offers valuable lessons for our modern world. By understanding how different foods influence our mental state and incorporating these insights into our daily lives, we can better support both our cognitive function and emotional well-being. This holistic approach to nutrition, viewing food as medicine for both body and mind, may be one of the most powerful tools we have for promoting longevity and maintaining mental vitality throughout our lives.

Cultural Rituals for Emotional Processing and Stress Release

Throughout human history, cultures have developed sophisticated rituals for processing emotions and releasing stress - practices that modern science now recognizes as crucial for both mental health and longevity[12] [26] [25]. From the social support networks of Okinawa's moai to the mindful meditation practices of Buddhist traditions, these time-tested approaches offer powerful tools for managing the emotional challenges that can accelerate aging and diminish quality of life.

In Okinawa, one of the world's most renowned longevity hotspots, the moai system stands as a testament to the power of ritualized social support[25]. These lifelong social groups provide both emotional and practical support to their members, creating a built-in system for processing life's challenges and celebrations. Research has shown that such strong social connections correlate with lower levels of stress hormones and improved immune function - both key factors in longevity[26][25].

The power of these cultural rituals lies in their ability to activate multiple pathways of stress reduction simultaneously. When members of an Ikarian community gather for their traditional festivals and shared meals, they're not just enjoying social connection - they're engaging in practices that lower blood pressure, reduce stress hormones, and strengthen emotional resilience[25]. These gatherings provide structured opportunities for laughter, storytelling, and emotional expression, all of which have been linked to improved mental health and increased lifespan[26][25].

Traditional Chinese Medicine offers another sophisticated approach to emotional processing through practices like Qigong and Tai Chi[80]. These movement-based rituals combine physical activity with focused intention, helping to release emotional blockages while promoting the flow of vital energy. Centenarians in China often credit these practices for their remarkable emotional equilibrium and stress resilience, highlighting the importance of mind-body integration in longevity[80].

Particularly noteworthy are the gratitude and storytelling rituals found across various cultures. These practices provide structured ways to process both positive and negative experiences, helping to build emotional resilience while strengthening social bonds. Research suggests that regular expression of gratitude and participation in communal storytelling correlates with reduced stress levels and increased life satisfaction among centenarians[26][80].

The physiological benefits of these cultural rituals are profound. Many involve elements of singing, chanting, or meditative movement, which activate the parasympathetic nervous system - our body's natural "rest and digest" mode[26][25]. This activation helps lower blood pressure, reduce stress hormones, and promote cellular repair mechanisms that support longevity. Additionally, the social cohesion fostered by these rituals provides a protective buffer against the negative health impacts of chronic stress[26][25].

Modern research has validated what these traditional practices have long understood - that emotional processing and stress management are crucial for cognitive health and longevity[12][26]. Regular participation in cultural rituals that support emotional well-being has been linked to reduced risk of cognitive decline and improved mental clarity well into advanced age[29]. These benefits appear to be particularly pronounced when rituals incorporate multiple elements - physical movement, social connection, and mindful awareness[26][80].

Perhaps most significantly, these cultural rituals offer something often missing in modern approaches to stress management - a sense of meaning and continuity. By connecting individuals to their cultural heritage and community, these practices provide a framework for understanding and processing life's challenges that goes beyond simple stress reduction[80]. This deeper sense of meaning and belonging has been identified as a crucial factor in the remarkable longevity observed in traditional communities[12][26][25].

As we continue to understand the mechanisms behind these practices, their value becomes increasingly clear. Whether through structured social support systems like the Okinawan moai, movement practices like Tai Chi, or communal gatherings that blend multiple elements of emotional processing, these cultural rituals offer time-tested approaches to managing stress and supporting longevity[12][26][80][25]. In our modern world, where chronic stress and emotional disconnection often seem inevitable, these ancient practices provide valuable templates for building more resilient and sustainable approaches to emotional well-being.As we conclude this exploration of the mind-body connection and its profound impact on longevity, we're reminded that the wisdom of our ancestors continues to find validation through modern scientific research. The traditional practices we've examined - from sophisticated breathing techniques to movement meditation and sound healing - offer practical tools for managing the unique stresses of contemporary life while promoting both healthspan and lifespan.

What's particularly striking is how these ancient approaches to stress management align with our modern understanding of the body's longevity mechanisms. The breathing practices that yogis developed thousands of years ago are now known to directly influence our nervous system, reducing inflammation and supporting cellular repair. The movement meditations like Tai Chi, which traditional societies integrated into daily life, have been shown to enhance both physical and cognitive function while reducing the impact of stress on our bodies.

Through Sophia's story, we witnessed how these traditional practices can be effectively adapted to modern contexts without losing their essential benefits. Her journey from overwhelmed ER nurse to balanced healthcare practitioner demonstrates the practical application of these ancient wisdom traditions in managing contemporary stress. Moreover, her experience shows how these practices can create ripple effects, extending their benefits beyond the individual to touch the lives of others.

The sound healing traditions we explored reveal another dimension of the mind-body connection - one that operates at the cellular level through vibrational resonance. These practices, combined with mindful movement and conscious breathing, create a comprehensive approach to stress management that supports our body's natural longevity pathways.

Perhaps most significantly, we've seen how traditional mind-body nutrition and cultural rituals for emotional processing provide frameworks for understanding the deep connection between mental state and physical health. These practices offer not just stress relief, but a more profound sense of meaning and connection that research increasingly shows is crucial for longevity.

As we move forward in our longevity journey, the key lies not in choosing between ancient wisdom and modern science, but in understanding how they complement each other. The stress management techniques developed by our ancestors provide a foundation that modern research continues to validate and explain. By incorporating these practices into our daily lives - whether through mindful breathing during a busy workday, regular movement meditation, or participation in cultural rituals - we can access powerful tools for extending both the length and quality of our lives.

The mind-body connection represents one of the most powerful levers we have for influencing our longevity. As we've seen throughout this chapter, traditional practices offer time-tested methods for managing this connection, while modern science helps us understand and optimize their benefits. By embracing this synthesis of old and new, we can build more resilient approaches to stress management and create the conditions for a longer, healthier life.

Remember, the journey to longevity isn't just about adding years to life, but about adding life to years. The mind-body practices we've explored offer pathways to both, helping us cultivate the mental clarity, emotional balance, and physical vitality that characterize the world's most successful centenarians. As we continue our exploration of longevity practices in the following chapters, keep in mind that the foundation for physical health often begins with the state of our minds and the wisdom of listening to our bodies.

CHAPTER 8

Your Personal Longevity Blueprint

Designing a Life of Purpose and Health

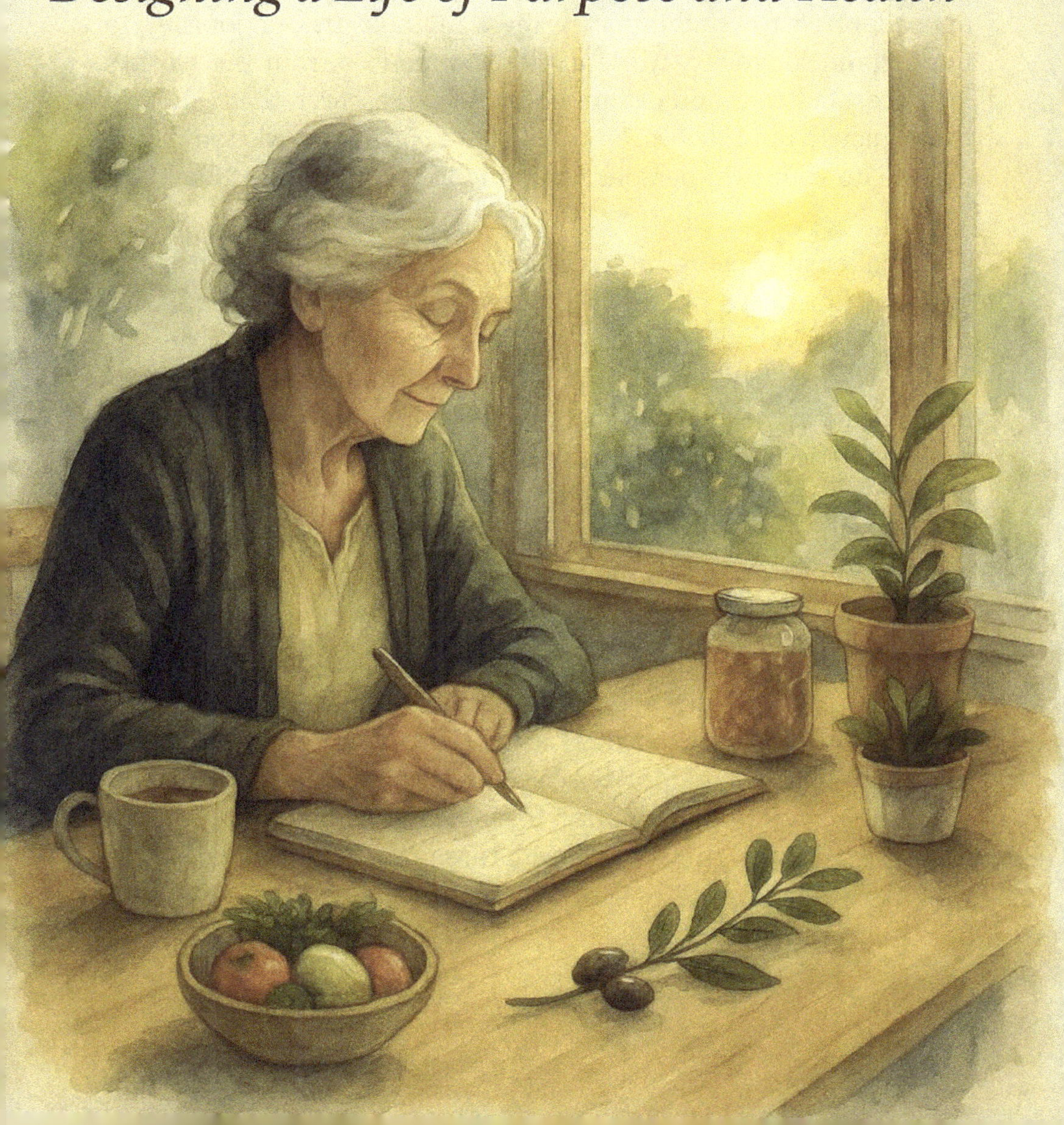

In the intricate tapestry of human health traditions, each thread of ancient wisdom carries profound relevance for our modern quest for longevity. The challenge lies not in choosing between old and new, but in weaving together a personalized blueprint that honors time-tested practices while embracing scientific advances and adapting to contemporary life demands. In our journey to understand longevity, we've explored practices from the world's healthiest cultures and examined scientific research that validates these ancient approaches. Now it's time to bring this wisdom home - to create your own personalized blueprint for a longer, healthier life.

The challenge of adapting traditional practices to modern life is perfectly illustrated by Amelia, a 42-year-old technology executive from Silicon Valley. Her story resonates deeply with the struggles many of us face in today's fast-paced world. Working 60-hour weeks in the heart of the tech industry, Amelia initially viewed traditional health practices as relics of the past, incompatible with her modern lifestyle. However, when faced with burnout and early signs of chronic health issues, she embarked on a journey that would transform her understanding of how ancient wisdom could be adapted for contemporary life.

Amelia's approach was methodical and practical. She identified three key traditional practices that addressed her most pressing needs: morning sun exposure - an ancient practice for regulating circadian rhythms, mindful tea ceremonies for stress management, and evening walking meditation for movement and mental clarity. Rather than attempting to replicate these practices exactly as they were performed centuries ago, she cleverly adapted them to fit her demanding schedule.

What made Amelia's story particularly compelling was her innovative approach to modernization. She programmed her smart home lighting to simulate dawn, creating a modern version of traditional sun exposure practices. Her office tea ceremony, though abbreviated to two minutes, maintained the essential elements of mindfulness and presence. Perhaps most ingeniously, she combined her evening walking meditation with conference calls, finding a way to honor both traditional wisdom and professional demands.

Over six months, these thoughtfully adapted practices led to measurable improvements in her wellbeing - better sleep patterns, reduced stress levels, and enhanced work performance. Her story teaches us a valuable lesson: successful adaptation of traditional practices isn't about perfect replication, but rather about understanding core principles and finding creative ways to apply them within modern constraints.

In this chapter, we'll explore how to create your own personalized longevity blueprint, one that honors both ancient wisdom and modern science while accounting for your unique circumstances. We'll provide practical frameworks for assessing your current health status, identifying relevant traditional practices, and adapting them to fit your lifestyle and goals. By understanding the fundamental principles behind these time-tested practices, you can craft sustainable habits that serve you well in today's world.

Whether you're a busy professional like Amelia, a parent juggling multiple responsibilities, or someone simply looking to age well, this chapter will guide you through the process of weaving traditional wisdom into the fabric of your modern life. Remember, the goal isn't to perfectly replicate ancient practices, but to harness their essential benefits in ways that work for you.

Personal Health Assessment: Traditional Diagnostic Methods Meet Modern Testing

Understanding our health status through both ancient wisdom and modern science provides a powerful framework for extending our lifespan far beyond what our ancestors could have imagined. In earlier centuries, when the average life expectancy hovered around 40 years, people relied solely on observational methods to assess their health - watching for changes in physical appearance, energy levels, and bodily functions. Today, we stand at an extraordinary intersection where these time-tested observational techniques can be combined with cutting-edge diagnostic tools to create a more complete picture of our health.

Traditional diagnostic methods, particularly those from Chinese Medicine and Ayurveda, offer profound insights into subtle bodily changes that might escape modern testing. These ancient systems recognize that our bodies provide early warning signs of imbalance long before disease manifests. For instance, Traditional Chinese Medicine practitioners assess the quality, rhythm, and strength of the pulse at different positions on the wrist, each believed to correspond to specific organ systems. Similarly, Ayurvedic doctors evaluate an individual's dosha (constitutional type) through detailed observation of physical characteristics and behavioral patterns.

Modern diagnostic testing brings precision and objectivity to health assessment through comprehensive blood panels, genetic testing, and advanced imaging[12]. These tools can detect disease markers and risk factors years before symptoms appear, allowing for early intervention. The real magic happens when we combine both approaches. For example, while a blood test might show normal thyroid levels, traditional pulse diagnosis might detect subtle energy imbalances that warrant preventive measures.

The integration of these approaches is particularly crucial for brain health, where both traditional wisdom and modern science emphasize the importance of early detection and prevention[29]. Traditional practices have long recognized the connection between lifestyle factors and cognitive vitality, while modern research validates these observations through neuroimaging and biochemical testing. Regular monitoring of both subjective experiences (memory, mood, mental clarity) and objective markers (inflammatory indicators, nutrient levels, brain volume) provides a comprehensive approach to maintaining cognitive health.

When creating your personal health assessment strategy, consider incorporating both traditional and modern methods[12]. Begin your day with a traditional self-assessment: observe your tongue coating, note your energy levels, and check your pulse quality. Complement these observations with regular modern health screenings, including comprehensive blood work, genetic testing, and age-appropriate preventive scans. This dual approach helps identify potential health issues from multiple angles, increasing the likelihood of early intervention.

The key to longevity lies not in choosing between traditional and modern methods, but in understanding how they complement each other. Traditional diagnostic techniques excel at detecting subtle imbalances and viewing the body as an interconnected system, while modern testing provides concrete data and early warning signs of specific conditions. Together, they create a more complete picture of health status and potential risks.

Remember that personal health assessment isn't just about identifying problems - it's about understanding your body's unique patterns and needs[11]. Regular monitoring through both traditional and modern means helps you recognize your baseline 'normal' and detect deviations early. This knowledge empowers you to make informed decisions about diet, exercise, stress management, and other lifestyle factors that influence longevity.

As you develop your personal health assessment routine, maintain detailed records of both traditional observations and modern test results. This documentation helps identify patterns over time and provides valuable information for both healthcare practitioners and traditional healers. Consider using modern technology to track traditional health markers - many apps now exist that help monitor pulse patterns, tongue appearance, and other traditional diagnostic indicators.

Customizing Ancient Practices for Your Lifestyle and Goals

The art of customizing ancient practices for modern life begins with understanding how human longevity has evolved over centuries. In earlier times, when life expectancy rarely exceeded 40 years, our ancestors faced challenges we've largely overcome through advances in medicine, sanitation, and nutrition. Yet the wisdom they developed for maintaining health and vitality remains remarkably relevant, especially when adapted thoughtfully to our contemporary context.[26][81]

The key to successful adaptation lies in understanding the core principles behind traditional practices rather than attempting to replicate them exactly. Consider the traditional practice of rising with the sun - while our ancestors did this by necessity, we now understand the scientific importance of morning light exposure for regulating circadian rhythms and supporting brain health[26]. Modern adaptations might include using dawn simulation lamps during winter months or scheduling morning walks to capture natural light, even if your workday starts later.

Brain health, in particular, benefits from a thoughtful fusion of ancient wisdom and modern science. Traditional practices like meditation, which centenarians have long credited for mental clarity, are now validated by neuroscience research showing their positive effects on brain structure and function[26][81]. The key is finding ways to incorporate these practices that align with your daily routine - perhaps starting with five minutes of mindful breathing during your morning commute or lunch break.

Nutritional practices from long-lived populations offer another area ripe for modern adaptation. While the traditional Okinawan diet is plant-based and rich in sweet potatoes, the essential principle is consuming nutrient-dense, minimally processed foods[26][81]. This can be adapted to any cultural context or food preference while maintaining the core benefits. For instance, if traditional fermented foods don't appeal to you, modern probiotic supplements might provide similar gut health benefits, though whole food sources remain ideal when possible.

Physical activity patterns from centenarian cultures demonstrate the importance of natural movement throughout the day rather than isolated exercise sessions[26][81]. While traditional societies achieved this through farming and daily chores, modern adaptations might include taking stairs instead of elevators, having walking meetings, or using a standing desk. The goal is to break up periods of sedentary behavior with movement, even if it looks different from our ancestors' routines.

Stress management techniques from various cultures can be particularly powerful when adapted thoughtfully[26][81]. Traditional practices like the Japanese forest bathing (shinrin-yoku) might be modified for urban environments by spending time in local parks or creating a nature-inspired space in your home. The essential element is regular connection with natural elements, even if they're adapted for city living.

Social connections, a cornerstone of longevity in traditional societies, require creative adaptation in our increasingly digital world[26]. While technology can't fully replace face-to-face interaction, it can help maintain meaningful connections when used intentionally. The key is ensuring that digital tools enhance rather than replace real-world relationships.

When customizing ancient practices, it's essential to consider your individual circumstances, including work schedule, family responsibilities, and living environment[81]. Start by identifying the core principles of traditional practices that resonate with you, then experiment with different adaptations until you find what works. Remember that consistency matters more than perfection - a simplified practice done regularly often yields better results than an elaborate routine attempted sporadically.

Measuring the effectiveness of your adapted practices is crucial[11]. While traditional societies relied on observation and experience, we can combine these with modern metrics like sleep quality data, stress markers, and cognitive assessments. This blend of subjective experience and objective measurement helps ensure your adaptations maintain the benefits of traditional practices.

Finally, remember that adaptation is an ongoing process[26][81][11]. As your life circumstances change, your practices may need to evolve. The goal is to create sustainable habits that honor ancient wisdom while fitting seamlessly into your modern lifestyle. This flexible approach, grounded in traditional principles but adapted for contemporary life, offers the best path to extending both lifespan and healthspan in today's world.

Creating Sustainable Daily Rituals: The Art of Habit Formation

The journey to a longer, healthier life begins with understanding how our ancestors approached daily routines and rituals. In earlier centuries, when life expectancy rarely exceeded 40 years, people's daily habits were primarily focused on immediate survival rather than long-term health. Today, we have the luxury of crafting intentional routines that can extend our lives well beyond what our ancestors could have imagined, thanks to advances in science and our deeper understanding of how habits shape our health[12][82].

Modern research validates what many centenarians have long practiced - the power of consistent, purposeful daily rituals. As James Clear, author of Atomic Habits, explains: "Every action you take is a vote for the type of person you wish to become. No single instance will transform your beliefs, but as the votes build up, so does the evidence of your new identity."[82] This insight perfectly captures the essence of how small, daily actions compound over time to create lasting health benefits.

The science behind habit formation reveals three core components that we must understand to create sustainable rituals: the cue (trigger), the routine (behavior), and the reward (benefit)[82]. When examining the daily practices of centenarians across Blue Zones - from Sardinia to Okinawa - we see these components naturally embedded in their cultural traditions[82]. Their habits aren't forced or artificial; they're seamlessly woven into the fabric of daily life.

Particularly crucial for longevity is the establishment of brain-healthy rituals. Research shows that cognitive decline isn't an inevitable part of aging but rather significantly influenced by our daily habits[26][12]. Centenarians often maintain sharp minds well past 100 through consistent mental stimulation, social engagement, and stress management techniques[26][12]. These practices help build cognitive reserve and protect against neurodegenerative diseases

To create sustainable daily rituals, start small and build gradually[82]. Dan Buettner, renowned longevity researcher, emphasizes: "The secret to longevity is not to try to change everything at once, but to make small changes that are easy to stick with for the rest of your life."[82] This might mean beginning with a five-minute morning meditation, then gradually extending the duration as the habit becomes ingrained.

Anchor new habits to existing routines - this is a powerful strategy used by many centenarians[82]. For example, in Okinawa, the practice of "ikigai" (finding one's purpose) is naturally integrated into daily activities, from tending gardens to participating in community gatherings[12]. Modern adaptations might include combining your daily walk with listening to educational podcasts or making family dinner a time for both nutrition and meaningful conversation.

The environment plays a crucial role in habit formation. Centenarians typically live in communities that naturally support healthy behaviors - from walkable neighborhoods to social structures that encourage regular interaction[26][12][82]. While we may not be able to replicate these exact conditions, we can modify our surroundings to support our chosen habits. This might mean keeping healthy snacks visible, creating a dedicated space for meditation, or organizing regular social activities with friends who share similar health goals.

Perhaps most importantly, sustainable rituals must be meaningful and enjoyable[26][12]. The longest-living populations don't view their healthy habits as burdensome - these practices are sources of pleasure and purpose. Whether it's sharing meals with loved ones, engaging in gentle morning movement, or participating in community activities, their health-promoting behaviors are intrinsically rewarding.

When developing your own longevity rituals, consider the preventative health practices that complement traditional wisdom[12]. Regular health screenings, stress management techniques, and proactive care form an essential modern habit framework that builds upon ancient knowledge. Remember that consistency matters more than perfection - it's better to maintain a simple daily walk than to attempt an unsustainable intensive exercise regime.

Measuring progress helps maintain motivation, but avoid becoming overly focused on immediate results. The power of daily rituals lies in their cumulative effect over time[26][12][82]. As demonstrated by centenarians worldwide, it's the small, consistent actions - performed day after day, year after year - that ultimately contribute to extraordinary longevity and vitality.

Environmental Adaptation: Traditional Wisdom for Modern Challenges

Throughout human history, our ancestors developed remarkable strategies for adapting to their environments, strategies that modern science is now validating as crucial for longevity[11][12]. In earlier centuries, when life expectancy hovered around 40 years, people faced numerous environmental challenges - from extreme weather conditions to limited food availability and poor sanitation. These harsh conditions, combined with insufficient medical knowledge and inadequate public health measures, contributed to shortened lifespans. Today, we have the opportunity to combine ancient environmental wisdom with modern scientific understanding to create optimal conditions for longevity.

The Blue Zones offer compelling evidence of how environmental adaptation influences lifespan[11][13]. In these regions - from Okinawa to Sardinia - centenarians have thrived by maintaining traditional practices that harmonize with their natural surroundings. They typically live in environments that encourage daily walking, gardening, and physical labor, naturally reducing sedentary behavior[11]. Their communities are structured to foster strong social bonds, with spaces designed for regular interaction and shared activities[11][12].

Jeanne Calment's remarkable life of 122 years in Arles, France, demonstrates how environmental adaptation can support exceptional longevity[11][13]. Living in a small Mediterranean town, she maintained daily walks, consumed locally sourced food, and remained socially engaged throughout her life. Her story illustrates that longevity isn't merely about genetics but about how we interact with our environment.

Brain health, in particular, benefits from traditional environmental wisdom. Centenarians often live in communities that naturally support cognitive vitality through regular social interaction, physical activity, and engagement with nature[11][12].

Modern neuroscience confirms that these environmental factors play crucial roles in preventing cognitive decline and maintaining mental acuity into advanced age[12].

The challenge for modern individuals lies in adapting these traditional environmental practices to contemporary settings[12]. While we may not all live in Blue Zones, we can implement key principles from these longevity-promoting environments. This might mean creating walking routes in urban areas, establishing community gardens in city spaces, or organizing regular social gatherings that mirror traditional community structures.

Diet represents another crucial area where environmental adaptation impacts longevity. Traditional societies understood the importance of eating locally available, seasonal foods[12] [13]. Modern research confirms that this approach not only provides optimal nutrition but also supports environmental sustainability. The Mediterranean and Okinawan diets, rich in locally grown vegetables, fruits, and legumes, offer proven templates for healthy eating that can be adapted to various geographical locations[12].

Stress management through environmental adaptation is another vital lesson from centenarian cultures[12]. Traditional practices often incorporate natural elements for stress reduction - from forest bathing in Japan to Mediterranean siesta cultures. These practices recognize the profound impact of environment on mental health and stress levels, a connection now supported by extensive scientific research[12].

Technology can play a role in modern environmental adaptation without compromising traditional wisdom[12]. While our ancestors relied on natural cues for timing daily activities, we can use smart devices to remind us to move regularly, spend time outdoors, or engage in social activities. The key is using technology to support rather than replace traditional environmental practices.

To create your own environmental adaptation strategy, start by assessing your current surroundings. Look for opportunities to incorporate more natural movement, social interaction, and connection with nature into your daily routine. Consider how traditional wisdom about seasonal eating, community engagement, and stress management can be adapted to your specific situation[12].

Remember that successful environmental adaptation isn't about perfectly replicating traditional living conditions - it's about understanding the principles behind these practices and finding modern equivalents. Whether you live in an urban apartment or a suburban house, you can create an environment that supports longevity by incorporating elements from centenarian cultures while acknowledging contemporary realities.

The integration of traditional environmental wisdom with modern science offers a powerful framework for extending both lifespan and healthspan[11] [12] [13]. By understanding how our ancestors adapted to their environments and applying these principles thoughtfully to our modern context, we can create living spaces and daily routines that naturally support longevity. This approach, combining ancient wisdom with contemporary knowledge, provides a sustainable path to healthier, longer lives in today's world.

Measuring Progress: Combining Traditional Markers with Modern Metrics

The journey to measure and optimize longevity has evolved dramatically from our ancestors' time, when reaching 40 was considered a remarkable achievement. In those earlier centuries, limited medical knowledge, poor sanitation, infectious diseases, and inadequate nutrition created a ceiling on human lifespan that seemed insurmountable. Today, we stand at an extraordinary intersection where traditional wisdom about longevity can be validated and enhanced through modern scientific metrics, offering unprecedented insights into how we age and how we can extend our healthspan.

Dr. Nir Barzilai's groundbreaking research has revealed how combining traditional markers with modern metrics can unlock powerful insights about longevity. His studies of centenarians and their offspring have demonstrated that certain biological markers, such as HDL cholesterol levels, can provide objective measurements of longevity potential. As he notes, "The HDL cholesterol of a centenarian was average...but their offspring had twice the HDL...That there's a longevity effect of HDL."[83] This discovery illustrates how modern metrics can validate and explain traditional observations about familial longevity.

Traditional markers of longevity often focused on observable qualities - energy levels, mobility, cognitive clarity, and social engagement[12]. These qualitative measures, while seemingly simple, have proven remarkably accurate in predicting healthy aging. Modern science now allows us to understand the biological mechanisms behind these traditional markers, providing quantifiable metrics through advanced testing methods like DNA methylation clocks, telomere length analysis, and epigenetic markers[83].

Particularly fascinating is the concept of "compression of morbidity" observed in centenarian populations. Research shows that many centenarians experience a significantly shorter period of illness at life's end compared to those who die younger. As Dr. Barzilai explains, "They were sick very little at the end of their lives."[83] This observation aligns with traditional wisdom about healthy aging while providing measurable metrics for modern health assessment.

Brain health monitoring represents a perfect example of how traditional markers and modern metrics can work together. While traditional societies recognized cognitive vitality through social engagement, memory retention, and problem-solving abilities, we now have sophisticated tools to track brain health through cognitive assessments, neuroimaging, and biomarker analysis[83]. This combination allows for early detection and intervention in cognitive decline, supporting the maintenance of mental acuity into advanced age.

Modern technology has revolutionized our ability to track health markers in real-time. Wearable devices monitor physical activity, sleep patterns, and heart rate variability, providing immediate feedback that our ancestors could only gauge through subjective experience[12]. These tools don't replace traditional wisdom but rather enhance our ability to implement and measure its effectiveness.

Preventative health practices, long emphasized in traditional longevity wisdom, can now be quantified and tracked with unprecedented precision. Regular screening for key health markers, combined with traditional preventative practices like stress management and dietary wisdom[12], creates a comprehensive approach to health monitoring that bridges ancient and modern understanding.

To effectively measure your progress toward optimal longevity, consider creating a personal dashboard that combines traditional markers with modern metrics. Track subjective measures like energy levels, mood, and social engagement alongside objective data from regular health screenings and wearable devices[12]. This integrated approach provides a more complete picture of your health trajectory than either method alone.

Remember that successful measurement of longevity progress isn't just about collecting data - it's about understanding what that data means in the context of your overall health and lifestyle. Regular review and adjustment of your health practices based on both traditional wisdom and modern metrics creates a dynamic, responsive approach to extending both lifespan and healthspan.

The future of longevity measurement lies in this synthesis of ancient wisdom and modern science. As we continue to develop more sophisticated tools for measuring biological age and health markers, we must remember to ground these measurements in the time-tested wisdom of traditional health practices. This balanced approach offers the best path forward for understanding and optimizing our journey toward healthy longevity.As we conclude this chapter on creating your personal longevity blueprint, it's remarkable to reflect on how far human longevity has come. Just two centuries ago, the average person could expect to live only 40 years, their life cut short by infectious diseases, poor sanitation, inadequate nutrition, and limited medical knowledge. Today, we stand at an extraordinary moment in human history where living past 100 isn't just possible - it's increasingly common in certain regions of the world.

Through our exploration of ancient wisdom and modern science, we've discovered that the path to exceptional longevity lies not in choosing between traditional and contemporary approaches, but in thoughtfully combining them. Amelia's story showed us how even the busiest professionals can adapt ancient practices to modern life without losing their essential benefits. Her success in incorporating morning light exposure, mindful tea ceremonies, and walking meditation demonstrates that small, consistent changes can lead to significant improvements in health and wellbeing.

The key principles we've covered - from personal health assessment to environmental adaptation - provide a framework for creating sustainable lifestyle changes that support longevity. We've learned that successful implementation isn't about perfect replication of traditional practices, but rather about understanding their core principles and finding creative ways to apply them within our modern constraints.

Particularly crucial is our understanding of brain health, where both traditional wisdom and modern science emphasize the importance of regular mental stimulation, social engagement, and stress management. These practices help build cognitive reserve and protect against neurodegenerative diseases, supporting mental clarity well into advanced age.

Remember that your longevity blueprint should be as unique as you are. While the principles we've discussed are universal, their application must be personalized to your circumstances, goals, and lifestyle. Start small, build gradually, and focus on consistency rather than perfection. Whether you're adapting traditional dietary wisdom, incorporating movement practices, or establishing stress management routines, choose modifications that you can maintain for the long term.

As you move forward with implementing your personal longevity blueprint, keep in mind that this is not a static document but a living, breathing guide that will evolve with you. Regular assessment and adjustment of your practices, using both traditional markers and modern metrics, will help ensure you're on the right path.

The journey to exceptional longevity is not about adding years to your life, but life to your years. By thoughtfully combining ancient wisdom with modern science, you can create a sustainable approach to health and vitality that serves you well into your later years. Remember, the practices that seem small today - the morning walks, the mindful meals, the moments of connection - compound over time to create extraordinary results.

Your personal longevity blueprint is more than just a collection of health practices - it's your roadmap to a longer, healthier, and more vibrant life. As you implement these strategies, you're not just following in the footsteps of centenarians; you're creating your own path to exceptional longevity, one that honors both traditional wisdom and modern science while remaining uniquely yours.

May your journey toward optimal health and longevity be filled with discovery, growth, and the joy of living well at every

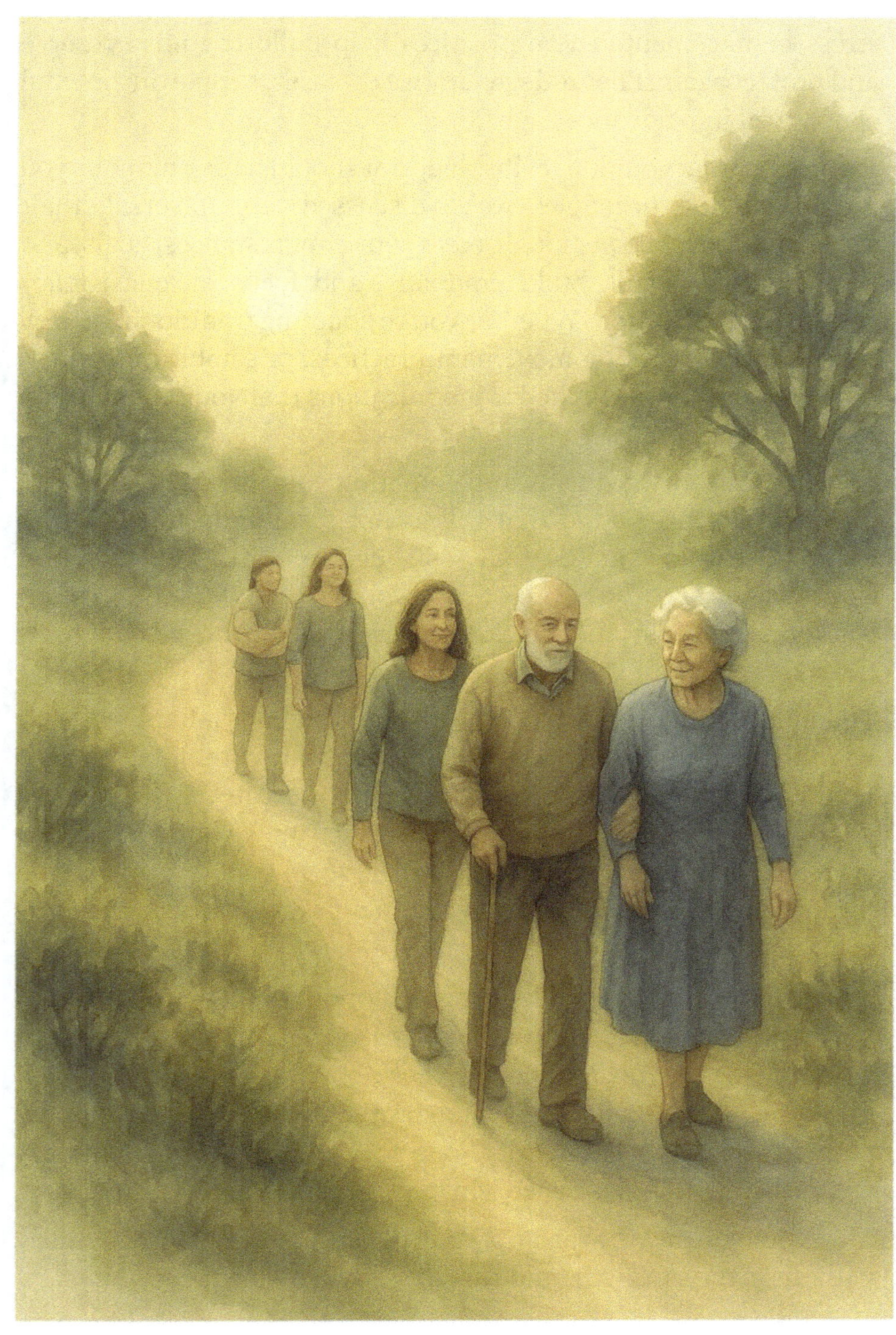

Conclusion

Often anticipate modern scientific findings. The emphasis on whole foods, natural movement, strong social connections, and stress management techniques has been validated by contemporary research, confirming what our ancestors somehow knew intuitively.

Particularly noteworthy is our deep dive into brain health, where we've seen how traditional practices like meditation, social engagement, and specific dietary patterns align perfectly with current neuroscientific understanding of cognitive preservation. The ancient practice of fermentation, once merely a means of food preservation, has been revealed by modern science as a crucial factor in gut health and overall longevity. These discoveries demonstrate how examining traditional practices through a scientific lens can uncover profound health benefits.

The dramatic increase in human lifespan over the past century isn't just due to medical advances and improved sanitation - though these have been crucial. It's also because we're beginning to understand and implement the wisdom of traditional cultures that have long maintained exceptional health well into advanced age. From the Blue Zones to the ancient healing traditions of various cultures, we've seen how lifestyle practices passed down through generations contain valuable insights for modern living.

Perhaps most importantly, we've learned that longevity isn't about following a rigid set of rules or completely abandoning modern life in favor of ancient practices. Instead, it's about understanding the principles behind these time-tested traditions and adapting them thoughtfully to our contemporary context. The personal stories we've shared throughout this book demonstrate how people from all walks of life have successfully integrated traditional wisdom into their modern routines, achieving remarkable improvements in their health and vitality.

As you move forward on your own longevity journey, remember that the goal isn't perfection but progress. Start with small, manageable changes that resonate with your lifestyle and gradually build upon them. Whether it's incorporating more fermented foods into your diet, practicing traditional movement patterns, or adopting stress-management techniques from ancient cultures, each step you take combines the wisdom of the past with the opportunities of the present.

The secrets of the centenarians aren't really secrets at all - they're time-tested practices that have proven their worth across generations and cultures. By understanding and adapting these practices while embracing the best of modern science, we can each create our own path to exceptional health and longevity. The journey to a longer, healthier life isn't just about adding years to our life - it's about adding life to our years.

As you close this book, remember that you now possess both ancient wisdom and modern knowledge to guide your choices. The potential for a long, vibrant life lies within your grasp. The centenarians have shown us the way - now it's our turn to follow in their footsteps while blazing our own trail toward exceptional health and longevity.

YOUR REVIEWS MATTER

Thank you for taking the time to read *Secrets of Centenarians*. This book was written with care, research, and deep respect for the wisdom of those who have lived long, meaningful lives.

If this book inspired you, taught you something new, or encouraged you to look at aging and longevity in a different way, your review truly matters.

Sharing your thoughts helps other readers discover this book and supports independent authors in continuing to create meaningful, research-driven work. Even a few honest sentences about what resonated with you can make a powerful difference.

Thank you for being part of this journey toward living longer, healthier, and more purpose-filled lives.

With gratitude,
Wendy D. Palmer

Bibliography

REFERENCES

1 Wikipedia contributors. (2024, February 23). *Hunter-gatherer.* Wikipedia, The Free Encyclopedia. https://en.wikipedia.org/wiki/Hunter-gatherer

2 Connor, T.. (2023, May). *The Myth that Hunter-Gatherers Didn't Live Long.* The Paleo Diet. https://thepaleodiet.com/myth-that-hunter-gatherers-didnt-live-long-bill-nye/

3 Spodek, J.. (2023). *Health and longevity of other cultures.* Joshua Spodek. https://joshuaspodek.com/health-and-longevity-of-other-cultures

4 Diamond, J.. (1987, May). *The Worst Mistake in the History of the Human Race.* Discover Magazine. https://web.cs.ucdavis.edu/~rogaway/classes/188/materials/diamond

5 Spencer Institute. (2023, June 23). *Exploring Human Longevity: A Journey Through Time and the Quest for Immortality.* Spencer Institute. https://spencerinstitute.com/exploring-human-longevity-a-journey-through-time-and-the-quest-for-immortality/

6 Desjardins, J.. (2020, May). *The world's rapid rise in life expectancy, visualized.* World Economic Forum. https://www.weforum.org/stories/2020/05/worlds-rise-life-expectancy-medicine-health/

7 Wosen, J.. (2024, October 07). *Wealthy nations might be reaching a life expectancy limit, study suggests — at least for now.* STAT News. https://www.statnews.com/2024/10/07/life-expectancy-reaches-limit-new-human-longevity-study-journal-nature-aging/

8 Goldman L.. (2018, January). *Three Stages of Health Encounters Over 8000 Human Generations and How They Inform Future Public Health.* American Journal of Public Health. https://pmc.ncbi.nlm.nih.gov/articles/PMC5719695/

9 Finch C. E.. (2009, December 4). *Evolution of the human lifespan and diseases of aging: Roles of infection, inflammation, and nutrition.* Proceedings of the National Academy of Sciences of the United States of America. https://pmc.ncbi.nlm.nih.gov/articles/PMC2868286/

10 Withington, J.. (2017, November). *Secrets of the Centenarians: What is it Like to Live for a Century and Which of Us Will Survive to Find Out?.* University of Chicago Press. https://press.uchicago.edu/ucp/books/book/distributed/S/bo27431957.html

11 GEW Social Sciences Group. (2024, June 1). *Decoding Longevity: Secrets Of The Centenarians.* Everand. https://www.everand.com/book/745948982/Decoding-Longevity-Secrets-Of-The-Centenarians

12 White, P.. (2023, October). *The Longevity Secrets of the Centenarians: What We Can Learn from the People Who Live the Longest.* ThriftBooks. https://www.thriftbooks.com/w/the-longevity-secrets-of-the-centenarians-what-we-can-learn-from-the-people-who-live-the-longest_peter-white/51355402/

13 Mickelson, C.. (2020, April 1). *Secrets of Longevity: Take the 30 Day Methuselah Challenge to Live Like a Centenarian.* Goodreads. https://www.goodreads.com/book/show/53595929-secrets-of-longevity

14 Buettner, D.. (2020, July). *Blue Zones Diet: Food Secrets of the World's Longest-Lived People.* Blue Zones. https://www.bluezones.com/2020/07/blue-zones-diet-food-secrets-of-the-worlds-longest-lived-people/

15 Buettner, D.. (2023, January 01). *Books.* Blue Zones. https://www.bluezones.com/books/

16 Buettner D.. (2016, July 7). *Blue Zones: Lessons From the World's Longest Lived.* American Journal of Lifestyle Medicine. https://pmc.ncbi.nlm.nih.gov/articles/PMC6125071/

17 Withington, J.. (2017, September 19). *Secrets of the Centenarians: What is it Like to Live for a Century and Which of Us Will Survive to Find Out?.* Barnes & Noble. https://www.barnesandnoble.com/w/secrets-of-the-centenarians-john-withington/1125899572

18 Day, J.. (2017, December 3). *5 Life Secrets That Centenarians Know.* Dr. John Day. https://drjohnday.com/5-life-secrets-that-centenarians-know/

19 Kiltro Team. (2024, September 21). *Blue Zones Social Connection: The Secret to Longevity and Well-being.* Kiltro Health. https://www.kiltrohealth.com/blog/blue-zones-social-connection-the-secret-to-longevity-and-well-being

20 Ikigai Kan. (2021, October). *Ikigai: The Japanese Secret to a Long and Happy Life - Book Review.* Ikigai Kan. https://ikigaikan.com/reviews/ikigai-the-japanese-secret-to-a-long-and-happy-life/

21 García H. & Miralles F.. (2018, January 01). *Ikigai: The Japanese Secret to a Long and Happy Life / The Little Book of Hygge / Lagom: The Swedish Art of Balanced Living.* Goodreads. https://www.goodreads.com/en/book/show/40534545-ikigai

22 De Felicis, J.. (2022, February). *13 Unusual Ways to Shed Stress (Lessons from the World's Blue Zones).* Blue Zones.

https://www.bluezones.com/2022/02/13-unusual-ways-to-shed-stress-lessons-from-the-worlds-blue-zones/

23 Collins, E.. (2025, June 20). *Longevity Secrets of Centenarians.* partiQlar. https://partiqlar.com/blogs/lifestyle/longevity-secrets-of-centenarians

24 Withington, J.. (2017, November 15). *Secrets of the Centenarians: What is it Like to Live for a Century and Which of Us Will Survive to Find Out?.* Goodreads. https://www.goodreads.com/en/book/show/34447893-secrets-of-the-centenarians

25 Khalsa D. S., Stauth C.. (1997, January 01). *Brain Longevity: The Breakthrough Medical Program that Improves Your Mind and Memory.* Goodreads. https://www.goodreads.com/book/show/1091982.Brain_Longevity

26 Ferguson, K.. (2023, May 08). *Longevity Secrets Of Centenarians.* The Centenarian Playbook. https://gemello.substack.com/p/longevity-secrets

27 Buck Institute. (2023, January 19). *The Secrets of Centenarians.* Buck Institute for Research on Aging. https://www.buckinstitute.org/podcasts/nir-barzilai-the-secrets-of-centenarians/

28 Sommerlad A., et al.. (2023, May 18). *Social participation and risk of developing dementia.* Nature Aging. https://www.nature.com/articles/s43587-023-00387-0

29 Felix, C. M.. (2020, October 19). *Regular Social Engagement Linked to Healthier Brain Microstructure in Older Adults.* The Gerontological Society of America. https://www.geron.org/News-Events/GSA-News/Press-Room/Press-Releases/regular-social-engagement-linked-to-healthier-brain-microstructure-in-older-adults

[30] Dodds L., Brayne C., Siette J.. (2024, March 4). *Associations between social networks, cognitive function, and quality of life among older adults in long-term care.* BMC Geriatrics. https://pmc.ncbi.nlm.nih.gov/articles/PMC10910782/

[31] Roth J. S.. (2023, January 25). *Social Activity, Aging Education Critical to Brain Health in Older African Americans, Study Finds.* BrightFocus Foundation. https://www.brightfocus.org/news/social-activity-aging-education-critical-brain-health-older-african-americans-study/

[32] Bennett, S.. (2025, September 16). *Ancient Sleep Wisdom: Why 68% of Adults Are Missing What I Discovered About Evening Relaxation.* Le Journal Catalan. https://www.le-journal-catalan.com/en/ancient-sleep-wisdom-why-68-of-adults-are-missing-what-i-discovered-about-evening-relaxation/

[33] Ancestral Kitchen. (2023, March 09). *Improve Your Sleep With Ancestral Wisdom.* Ancestral Kitchen. https://ancestralkitchen.com/2023/03/09/improve-your-sleep-with-ancestral-wisdom/

[34] Arrazati, D. G.. (2024, March 19). *Liver King's 9 Ancestral Tenets for Health and Longevity: Science or Fad?.* NAD.com. https://www.nad.com/news/liver-kings-9-ancestral-tenants-for-health-and-longevity-science-or-fad

[35] Zeng, A.. (2025, February 20). *Nighttime Eating and Longevity: What Ancient Wisdom and Modern Science Agree On.* Karviva. https://karviva.com/2025/02/20/nighttime-eating-and-longevity-what-ancient-wisdom-and-modern-science-agree-on/

[36] The Healthline Editorial Team. (2025, March 13). *8 Fermented Foods and Drinks to Boost Digestion and Health.* Healthline. https://www.healthline.com/nutrition/8-fermented-foods

37 Davis, J.. (2025, February 27). *Benefits of Fermented Foods.* WebMD. https://www.webmd.com/diet/ss/slideshow-benefits-fermented-foods

38 American Medical Association. (2025, September 24). *From kimchi to kefir: What to tell patients about fermented foods.* AMA News Wire. https://www.ama-assn.org/public-health/prevention-wellness/kimchi-kefir-what-tell-patients-about-fermented-foods

39 Bilodeau K.. (2023, September 12). *Fermented foods for better gut health.* Harvard Health Publishing. https://www.health.harvard.edu/blog/fermented-foods-for-better-gut-health-201805161607

40 Bieber A. M.. (2025, August 28). *The Health Benefits of Fermented Foods, From Kimchi to Kefir.* Cedars-Sinai Blog. https://www.cedars-sinai.org/blog/the-health-benefits-of-fermented-food-from-kimchi-to-kefir.html

41 Weaver, J.. (2021, July 12). *Fermented-food diet increases microbiome diversity, decreases inflammatory proteins, study finds.* Stanford Medicine News. https://med.stanford.edu/news/all-news/2021/07/fermented-food-diet-increases-microbiome-diversity-lowers-inflammation.html

42 Ludwig D. S.. (2021, April 19). *Fermented foods can add depth to your diet.* Harvard Health Publishing. https://www.health.harvard.edu/staying-healthy/fermented-foods-can-add-depth-to-your-diet

43 SmartSense. (2018, July 4). *Food Safety Milestones Part 1: A Short History of Food Preservation.* SmartSense Blog. https://blog.smartsense.co/short-history-of-food-preservation

44 Nummer B. A.. (2002, May). *Historical Origins of Food Preservation.* National Center for Home Food Preservation. https://nchfp.uga.edu/resources/entry/historical-origins-of-food-preservation

45 MadgeTech Marketing. (2021, November 16). *7 Ancient Methods of Food Preservation*. MadgeTech Blog. https://www.madgetech.com/posts/blogs/7-ancient-methods-of-food-preservation/

46 Dealy, A.. (2013, August 30). *Early Food Preservation in the Finger Lakes*. Historic Geneva. https://historicgeneva.org/food-and-cooking/early-food-preservation-in-the-finger-lakes/

47 Knez E., Kadac-Czapska K., Grembecka M.. (2023, February 27). *Effect of Fermentation on the Nutritional Quality of the Selected Vegetables and Legumes and Their Health Effects*. Life (Basel). https://pmc.ncbi.nlm.nih.gov/articles/PMC10051273/

48 Coyle, D.. (2023, July 13). *What Is Fermentation? The Lowdown on Fermented Foods*. Healthline. https://www.healthline.com/nutrition/fermentation

49 Chris Kresser. (2022, March 15). *The 13 Benefits of Fermented Foods and How They Improve Your Health*. Chris Kresser. https://chriskresser.com/the-13-benefits-of-fermented-foods-and-how-they-improve-your-health/

50 Cook, C., Ponder, M. A., & Strawn, L. K.. (2022, September 21). *Making Safe Fermented Foods and Beverages*. Virginia Cooperative Extension. https://www.pubs.ext.vt.edu/content/pubsextvt_edu/en/FST/fst-435/fst-435.html

51 Clean Food Living. (2024, January). *The 5 Safety Guidelines When Fermenting Vegetables*. Clean Food Living. https://cleanfoodliving.net/safety-guidelines-when-fermenting-vegetables/

52 Bartter, A.. (2025, August 19). *8 best longevity exercises to boost your lifespan, according to experts*. Marie Claire UK. https://www.marieclaire.co.uk/life/health-fitness/best-longevity-exercises

53 Well+Good Editors. (2023, July 22). *7 Functional Fitness Moves for Longevity That Keep Your Body Moving Comfortably*

as You Age. Well+Good. https://www.wellandgood.com/fitness/functional-fitness-moves-longevity

54 Prof. Jin-Xiong She. (2025, February 13). *7 Anti-Aging Exercises for Longevity (and One Workout to Avoid).* Jinfiniti. https://www.jinfiniti.com/anti-aging-exercises/

55 Fit and Well Staff. (2024). *Everyone should learn to master these six longevity-boosting exercises, according to an expert trainer.* Fit and Well. https://www.fitandwell.com/exercise/strength-workouts/everyone-should-learn-to-master-these-six-longevity-boosting-exercises-according-to-an-expert-trainer

56 Preiato D.. (2021, February 22). *Farmer's Walk: Benefits, Techniques, and Muscles Worked.* Healthline. https://www.healthline.com/nutrition/farmers-walk-benefits

57 Ahern, S.. (2025, April 23). *Why Farmers Walks Are One of the Most Effective Full-Body Workouts.* Big Money Methods. https://www.bigmoneymethods.com/p/why-farmers-walks-are-one-of-the-most-effective-full-body-workouts

58 Barragree R. and Busch C.. (2024, May 26). *Embracing Longevity: The Crucial Role of Farmer's Carries and Grip Strength in Aging Well.* WildHawk Physical Therapy. https://wildhawkphysicaltherapy.com/grip-strength-aging-well-farmers-carries/

59 Fit and Well Staff. (2024). *Don't miss these.* Fit and Well. https://www.fitandwell.com/features/this-is-the-one-move-we-should-all-be-doing-to-futureproof-our-bodies-says-an-expert-trainer

60 MTNTOUGH. (2023, September 5). *The Top 5 Farmer's Walk Benefits for Mountain Athletes.* MTNTOUGH. https://mtntough.com/blogs/mtntough-blog/farmer-walk-benefits

[61] Barlow, R.. (2024, February 21). *The Secrets of Living to 100*. Boston University. https://www.bu.edu/articles/2024/the-secrets-of-living-to-100/

[62] The Supportive Care. (2024, January). *How Breathing Techniques Help Calm the Nervous System*. The Supportive Care. https://www.thesupportivecare.com/blog/how-breathing-techniques-help-calm-the-nervous-system

[63] Asaad, H.. (2025, March 04). *How Breathing Techniques Influence Brain Function and Nerve Health*. Lone Star Neurology. https://lonestarneurology.net/others/how-breathing-techniques-influence-brain-function-and-nerve-health/

[64] Zaccaro A.. (2018, September 07). *How Breath-Control Can Change Your Life: A Systematic Review on Psycho-Physiological Correlates of Slow Breathing*. Frontiers in Human Neuroscience. https://www.frontiersin.org/journals/human-neuroscience/articles/10.3389/fnhum.2018.00353/full

[65] Yilmaz Balban M.. (2023, January 10). *Brief structured respiration practices enhance mood and reduce physiological arousal*. Cell Reports Medicine. https://pmc.ncbi.nlm.nih.gov/articles/PMC9873947/

[66] Sauer, M.. (2024, September 27). *10 Ways Tai Chi Can Benefit Your Health*. Healthline. https://www.healthline.com/health/tai-chi-benefits

[67] McPhillips, K.. (2024, October 26). *Tai chi isn't just for seniors. The workout boosts strength, flexibility, and longevity, no matter what your age*. Fortune. https://fortune.com/well/article/tai-chi-benefits-strength-flexibility-longevity/

[68] Du, Arthur. (2012, May). *Longevity and Tai Chi Quan*. Arthur Tai Chi. https://arthurtaichi.com/articles/310-2/

[69] The University of Kansas Health System. (2023). *The Health Benefits of T'ai Chi*. The University of Kansas Health System.

https://www.kansashealthsystem.com/health-resources/turning-point/programs/resilience-toolbox/tai-chi

[70] Rejuve.AI Team. (2023, October 6). *The Science of Sound: How Music and Frequency Impact Longevity.* Rejuve.AI. https://blog.rejuve.ai/the-science-of-sound-how-music-and-frequency-impact-longevity-abc9373e306b

[71] Neumann, J.. (2023, June 24). *The Science Behind Sound Healing: How Vibrations Can Improve Your Health.* Courageous Life Counseling. https://www.courageouslifecounseling.com/blog/2025/6/22/the-science-behind-sound-healing-how-vibrations-can-improve-your-health

[72] Goldsby T. L.. (2016, September 30). *Effects of Singing Bowl Sound Meditation on Mood, Tension, and Well-being: An Observational Study.* Journal of Evidence-based Complementary & Alternative Medicine. https://pmc.ncbi.nlm.nih.gov/articles/PMC5871151/

[73] Lawrenson, A.. (2025, September 21). *The rise of sound healing and how it can improve your wellbeing.* Rituals Magazine. https://www.rituals.com/en-us/mag-rituality-what-is-sound-healing.html

[74] Botta, Mary. (2023, April 08). *5 Surprising Scientific Benefits of Sound Healing.* Mary Botta. https://marybotta.com/2023/04/08/5-surprising-scientific-benefits-of-sound-healing/

[75] Ni, Maoshing. (2006, May 4). *Secrets of Longevity: Hundreds of Ways to Live to Be 100.* Goodreads. https://www.goodreads.com/book/show/312796.SecretsofLongevity

[76] Whiting, K.. (2021, September). *What's the secret to Okinawa's long life expectancy? 6 longevity tips from Japan's longest-living people.* World Economic Forum.

https://www.weforum.org/stories/2021/09/japan-okinawa-secret-to-longevity-good-health/

77 Kyla. (2025, January 2). *The Longevity Blueprint: Daily Habits to Help You Live to 100 and Beyond.* Kyla.com. https://kyla.com/p/blog/the-longevity-blueprint-daily-habits-to-help-you-live-to-100-and-beyond/

78 Fitzgerald, K.. (2025, August 19). *Why Centenarians Are Defying Science: Secrets to Living 100+.* Dr. Kara Fitzgerald. https://www.drkarafitzgerald.com/2025/08/19/nir-barzilai-longevity-aging/